The Other Princess Diane –

A Story of Valiant Perseverance

Against Medical Odds

Burton A. Waisbren, Sr., M.D., FACP

Order this book online at www.trafford.com
or email orders@trafford.com

Most Trafford titles are also available at major online book retailers.

Printed in Victoria, BC, Canada.

ISBN: 978-1-4269-2504-7 (soft)
ISBN: 978-1-4269-2534-4 (hard)

Library of Congress Control Number: 2010901156

*Our mission is to efficiently provide the world's finest, most comprehensive book publishing
service, enabling every author to experience success. To find out how to publish your book, your
way, and have it available worldwide, visit us online at www.trafford.com*

Trafford rev. 2/26/2010

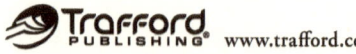 www.trafford.com

North America & international
toll-free: 1 888 232 4444 (USA & Canada)
phone: 250 383 6864 ✦ fax: 812 355 4082

DEDICATION

This book is dedicated to Diane and her family, but also to my wife and the physicians who made this possible.

About Dr. Waisbren

Dr. Burton Waisbren was born in Milwaukee, Wisconsin. He received his MD degree at the University of Wisconsin's Medical school, interned at the Harvard Service at the Boston City Hospital, served two years in the Navy at the Navy Research Institute in Bethesda and at the Biological Warfare Center in Frederick, Maryland, and was a resident and faculty member at the University of Minnesota Medical School in Minneapolis. He started a practice in his home town of Milwaukee in 1952 where he became a clinical associate professor at the Marquette University Medical school and then at the Medical College of Wisconsin Medical School. He was in charge of the infectious disease program at the Medical College from 1952 to 1970 and also became the Associate Medical Director of the St. Mary's Burn Center in Milwaukee in 1962.

He now practices in the office of his son, Dr. Charles Waisbren, where he can be reached through his website Waisbrenclinic@Ameritech.net and 414-771-5900.

AUTHOR'S ACKNOWLEDGEMENT

I am grateful to my brilliant daughter, Laura Stern, for her diligent assistance, loyal support, and painstaking proof-reading. Without her help, this book would not have been possible. All mistakes are my own, however.

Table of Contents

PROLOGUE

To help the non-medical reader understand what is described in this book this prologue will explain just what The Tetralogy of Fallot and Bacterial Endocarditis are.

The Tetralogy of Fallot

Fallot, a French surgeon first described this congenital heart syndrome in the late 19th century. In this syndrome a baby is born who appears blue (the blue baby syndrome). He/she is blue because the outflow valve of the right heart pump impedes the flow of blood as it tries to go into the lungs where it is suppose to pick up its oxygen. Because of this obstruction to the outlet of this pump (the right ventricle), pressure builds up in this pump. Because of this the blood forces its way through the membrane that separates the right ventricle from the pump that pumps the oxygenated blood to the entire body. The blood that is forced through this opening is blue because it has not been oxygenated in the lungs. The blue blood then turns the body blue. Hence the name blue baby syndrome became the name of this condition.

Dr. Potts, a pediatric surgeon at the Children's Hospital in Chicago, devised an operation that led to the extension of the lives of blue babies. In this operation he connected the aorta, the main artery of the body, to the artery that brings unoxygenated blood to the lungs. This bypassed the blocked valve of the right ventricle that blocked the unoxygenated blood from reaching the lungs. When the blood received oxygen in the lungs it was returned to the left ventricle from where it was then sent into the body.

Bacterial Endocarditis

In this disease, a bacterium sets itself up somewhere within the heart. From there, the heart pumps living organisms out to the entire body's organs where the bacteria multiply. The patient finally dies because the bacteria multiply in vital organs. This disease was invariably fatal until the early 1940s when it was found that penicillin could be given to the patient and that it could kill the bacteria and save the patient's life. During the time after 1940, it was found that some bacteria were not killed by penicillin. Then, when they multiply in many organs, they eventually kill the patient. It was bacteria of this type that caused Diane's problem.

INTRODUCTION

Readers who approached this book expecting it to be about the Princess who lived her life as a fairy tale will be in for a surprise. Rather, this book is about a courageous woman, Diane Cummings, who was the first person with the Tetralogy of Fallot to be operated upon by Dr. Willis J. Potts in 1946.* He was the pioneer surgeon who developed an operation for this syndrome in infants too young to have the operation that was reported before that time by Drs. Blalock and Trussing.

Diane went on to lead a full life while subsequently undergoing four more open-heart operations done by leaders in the field of the repair of the Tetralogy of Fallot who came after Dr. Potts. For this to have happened, she survived four episodes of subacute bacterial endocarditis due to unusual bacteria. She died in January 2007, having lived a full life for 62 years. This made her one of the longest survivors on record of Potts' original operation. This is her story.

Much of this story occurred after her endocarditis in 1962. She was fortunate to be treated by a series of doctors who have been and still are the pioneers in the development of corrective congenital heart disease. The reader will meet these outstanding physicians and read about their involvement with Diane. The doctors are Dr. Willis J. Potts of Children's Hospital in Chicago, the originator of the Potts' operation, the father and son team of Drs. James and John Kirklin who were at the University of Alabama Heart Center, and Dr. Joseph Dearani of the Mayo Clinic. The other main players were myself, Dr. McQuiston who was the anesthesiologist at the first operation, Dr. Joseph Noble, and the doctors Johnson, the husband and wife team who treated her fourth case of bacterial endocarditis.

My involvement with Diane started in 1962 when I was called in to treat her first case of endocarditis. She was an inspiration to me during the remaining forty-five years of her life.

*This narrative would not have been possible without the efforts and cooperation of Stephen Cummings, Diane's husband during most of her life.

CHAPTER ONE – Dr. Potts' First Operation for the Tetralogy of Fallot, 1946

Diane was born on December 10, 1943. It was apparent at birth that she had the congenital heart disease called the Tetralogy of Fallot (the blue baby syndrome) from the moment of her birth. Her parents lived in Waukesha, Wisconsin which is a small Wisconsin town about 30 miles west of Milwaukee. Her father was an energetic, loveable bear of a man who was involved in the brewery business in Waukesha. Her mother was a loving, warm woman who looked forward to being a "stay-at-home" mother. The parents were told from the beginning that at that time, blue babies rarely survived for more than a few years. Indeed that seemed to be the case since from the beginning, Diane failed to thrive. She could barely sit up and had periods of mild convulsions several times a day. Both parents were determined to do everything possible to help their tiny, non-thriving child but their efforts seemed to be in vain. However, Diane struggled on with constant loving attention from both parents.

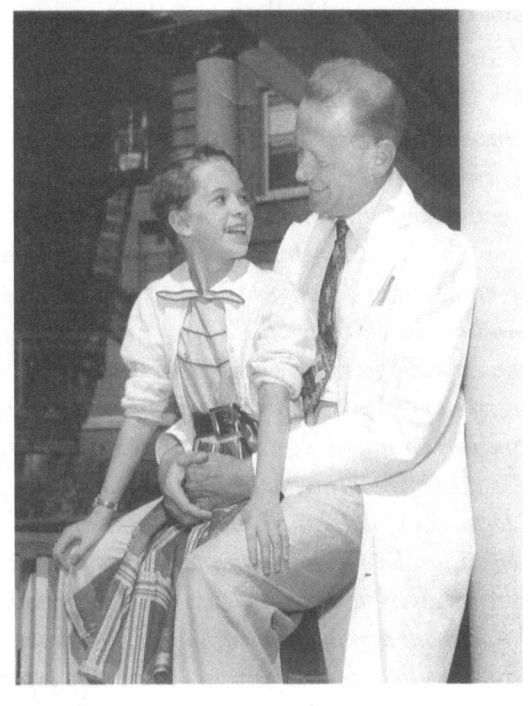

When she was 18 months old, her mother heard at the bridge table that there was a doctor at Children's Memorial Hospital in Chicago who was trying to develop a surgical cure for blue babies. She told her husband about this and within that week, Diane, her mother, her father, and Dr. Martin

Werra, her family doctor, went to see the doctor they had heard about. Dr. Potts* was not at the Children's Hospital at the time but someone at the desk gave Dr. Potts' home address to her parents. The family then drove to the Potts' home where Dr. Potts was cutting his grass.

*Dr. Potts retired in 1964 after many years as the chief pediatric surgeon at Children's Memorial Hospital in Chicago and as a professor of surgery at Northwestern University Medical School. He received the William E. Ladd Award in 1962 from the American Academy of Pediatrics.

What follows is an article that Dr. Potts wrote in the Reader's Digest in November of 1964. This article will give the reader some idea regarding the type of man Dr. Potts was. It was entitled, *We Gave Diane Back Her Life*, by Willis J. Potts, M.D.*

At first meeting, Andrew and Jane Schnell of Waukesha, Wisconsin, seemed unexceptional people. He was a businessman in his early 30's, prematurely gray; she, warm and outgoing, but with the subdued tension inevitable in a mother consulting one more in a long string of doctors, about a sick child.

*And Diane, their daughter, **was** sick, mortally sick. She was twenty-one months old and weighed only 18 pounds: a frail, longish child, all bones, and her whole body blue as watered grape juice. She was unable to sit up without support. Any excitement or exertion – even laughing, or crying, or eating too fast – sent her off into unconsciousness because the heart deformity she was born with kept sufficient oxygen from reaching her brain.*

Over the bridge table, of all places, her parents had heard that two doctors at Children's Memorial Hospital in Chicago were developing a new operation for the smallest and frailest of "blue babies". The Schnells had driven all the way from Waukesha on September 9, 1946, and I took Diane in without an appointment to see Dr. Stanley Gibson, our famed children's cardiologist. He brought them to the two experimenters: my colleague, Dr. Sidney Smith, and myself. And now Mrs. Schnell's eyes were pleading, Do you think you can do anything for our daughter?"

Even while Dr. Gibson and I were examining her, the little girl fainted dead away. We hurriedly ordered an emergency oxygen tent, but Mrs. Schnell quietly reassured us, "It's all right. She'll come out of it. This happens five or six times a day."

* This article must have been written before Dr. Potts heard about Diane's first case of endocarditis.

Diane did come around promptly, and Dr. Gibson and I breathed easier. It was the only occasion in my whole medical experience when the mother of a desperately sick child reassured me.

Mrs. Schnell came back to the point. "Now about this operation..."
I told them what I could do. "Yes, Dr. Smith and I were developing an operation for just such children as Diane. But so far we've done it only on dogs. We think it should work with a child, but we can't really be sure."

"Dogs? Just on dogs?" Mrs. Schnell asked. She hesitated, and for a long moment she and her husband merely looked at each other. Then she said, "The only other answer we've had from medical science is to take Diane home and make her life as happy as possible, because it's going to be a short one. We'd like to ask you, won't you try the operation on Diane?"

We admitted the child to the hospital for further examinations. Dr. Gibson, my co-worker and I told the Schnells that, "Yes, we thought the operation which up to that time had only been done on dogs would work, but if it was going to be done it had better be done quickly. Someday she was not going to come out of one of her spells."

I said I'd think it over. That night was for me a long and troubled one. True, the dogs had survived the operation – but they were healthy to begin with. Wasn't this child too frail to survive, to live? But then, she was already dying. Without the operation, she had no chance at all.

Next morning, I met with the Schnells again and explained the risks in some detail. I even drew them some sketches of the operation, which they studied silently. "It isn't perfect," I said. "It doesn't correct the deformities in the heart. It's designed to enable the patient to live, that's all. Do you still want to go ahead?"

They nodded. "Our minds are made up," Mrs. Schnell said to me. "Diane is a very poor surgical risk. So if you operate and she survives that will be proof that the operation will work."

"All right," I said, "tomorrow is Wednesday, we will operate in two days, on Friday morning."

The year before doctors Alfred Blalock and Helen B. Taussig at Johns Hopkins had taken a giant step toward solving the problem of the 'blue baby'. By bypassing leaky heart valves and constricted lung arteries, they severed the subclavian artery which leads to the child's arm and connected it to a lung artery instead. This extra channel shunted more blood to the lungs. This relieved the lack of oxygen that causes the blue baby syndrome. Because at under two years of age, a child's subclavian artery is often too small to serve this purpose, this operation could not be done on babies of Diane's age.

I wondered if in these cases it might not be possible to connect a lung artery to the side of the aorta itself. The main artery or 'river of life' that curves up out of the heart's left side. Medical experts agreed that such a connection would work, but they considered the feat impossible. Laboratory practice on dogs showed me that I needed at least 20 minutes to occlude, slit and sew together the two arteries. But clamping off a child's main artery and bloodstream for even less time than that will cause brain damage, paralysis or death.

I concluded I would have to pinch off a bit of the side wall of the aorta **without** impeding the flow in the bloodstream. But how? A baby's aorta, besides throbbing with every heartbeat, is as thin and slippery as a tube of wet macaroni. Every clamp I fashioned to do the job slipped off when we tried it on animals.

It was Dr. Smith who finally came up with an effective clamp that encircled the slippery aorta, cradling it, so that a workable fold of tissue could be pinched off. Using this clamp, Dr. Smith and I had performed thirty successful operations on dogs. But we were still refining our techniques when the Schnells appeared with Diane.

Now it was 9:00 a.m., September 13, 1946. The girl's thin, little body lies before me on the operating table, breathing softly under a light anesthetic. I could feel the tension myself and sense it in the nurses and doctors gathered in the operating room. Dr. Smith broke it with, "Chief, remember you've done this operation thirty times already." As I began the incision under the left armpit, my anxiety vanished with the need to concentrate.

The incision complete, I lifted the aorta and saw trouble. A startling network of at least a dozen small arteries branched off the aorta at the very spot where our clamp was to go. These were nature's own effort to compensate for Diane's inadequate heart. Each one would have to be ligated and cut before we could progress. Instead of a 30-minute operation, it would be a long one now.

Two hours later we had finished with those small arteries. Thanks to the efforts of expert anesthetist, Dr. William McQuiston, Diane was still breathing lightly and steadily. And now events seemed to turn our way. We tied off the pulmonary artery and applied our clamps to the aorta. It held perfectly. In each of the two vessels we made a precise lengthwise cut, one sixth of an inch, then joined the two slits together with fine silk thread.

After the suturing, we untied the pulmonary artery and slowly released the clamp on the side of the aorta. I had my fingers on the connection and *felt it throb now with the new flow of blood into the pulmonary artery. The results became apparent as slowly miraculously, Diane's color began to turn from blue to a rosy hue. Dr. Smith and I looked at each other, we didn't try to tell each other how we felt – there were no words adequate.*

Later Dr. Werra, the Schnells' family doctor who had been present in the operating room, took me aside to report the instructions Mrs. Schnell had given him that morning: "If Diane died on the operating table, I was to tell you to complete the operation to give you the experience that might help another child. I can only offer a silent salute to the deep love and perception of parents like that.

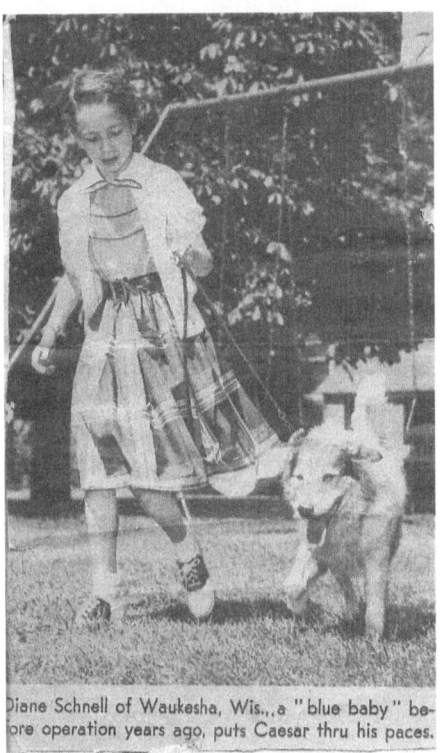

Diane Schnell of Waukesha, Wis.,,a " blue baby " before operation years ago, puts Caesar thru his paces.

At noon, Diane was wheeled out of the operating room. I went downstairs with her. Mr. and Mrs. Schnell jumped from their chairs and stared at their baby. In unison they cried, "Look, she's pink!"

We placed Diane in an oxygen tent as a precautionary measure. She improved each day. By the nineteenth day, she was almost like a normal child, and the Schnells took her home. There she skipped the crawling stage, got up on her feet and started to learn to walk.

Our prayers had been answered. Today at nineteen, Diane is a lively, bright young lady with laughing brown eyes. She swims, dances, bicycles and leads a normal life.

Every year on September 16, our anniversary, I telephone her and we have a chat. Sometimes I use the nickname her classmates gave her which was "Dynamite".

When one reads Dr. Potts' writings, his humanity and love for children stand out. His brilliance is evident when one reads the account of Diane's operation, which was just presented.

After the operation described by Dr Potts in Readers Digest Diane became for all intents and purposes, a normal child. She was very popular and as her sister put it, "beloved", as she kept up with the boisterous family activities with the brother and sister. Dr. Potts, true to his work, called Diane and her parents annually on the anniversary of her surgery which was done September 16, 1946, to see how she was getting along and to convey his good wishes. Diane and her parents reciprocated by accepting Dr. Potts' invitation to come to New York some years later to address a group of hospital administrators and doctors who were starting a pediatric surgical department. She told those at the meeting what the operation had meant to her.

CHAPTER TWO – First Bout of Staphylococcal Endocarditis Treated in Milwaukee, 1962

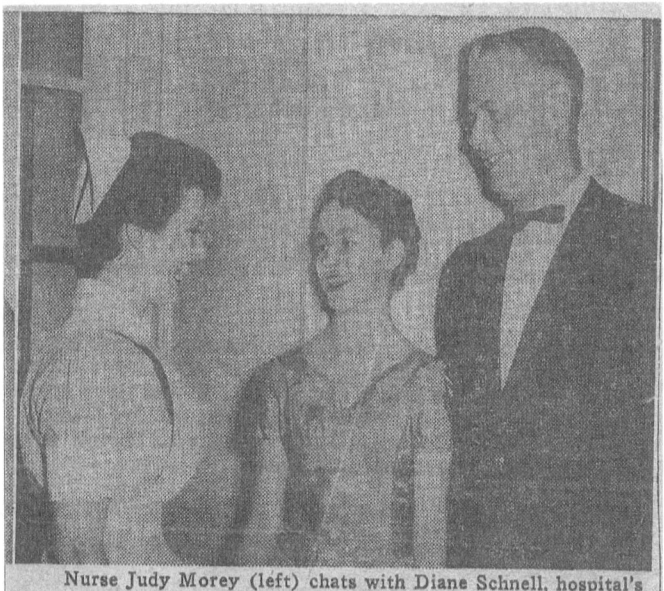

Nurse Judy Morey (left) chats with Diane Schnell, hospital's first blue baby, and her father Andrew Schnell, who attended black tie dinner for 5¼ million dollar program.

Shortly after Diane received her annual call from Dr. Potts in September of 1962, she began to run a daily fever. Dr. Werra, the family doctor who had originally gone with the Schnells to see Dr. Potts and who had observed the original operation, hospitalized Diane at Waukesha Memorial Hospital in Waukesha, Wisconsin. Waukesha is a town that then had a population of about 40,000, and is located thirty miles from Milwaukee. Diane became acutely ill and had several blood cultures that were positive for a coagulase positive staphylococcus which was resistant to the Penicillin. To complicate matters, Diane had developed a generalized rash from either Penicillin or Erythromycin that had been her initial therapy. She became increasingly ill, febrile, and hypertensive. I do not remember if Dr. Werra had been a student of mine who had heard me lecture to the students at the Marquette School of Medicine or whether he had had me consult on other of his patients. At any rate, he told the Schnells that he was stumped and wanted me to see Diane in consultation. He called me with the information that Diane was running a high fever, had a low blood pressure and seemed to be lapsing into a coma. I was making teaching rounds at the Milwaukee County Hospital at this time. I ended the rounds and drove to Waukesha Memorial Hospital, and indeed Diane was acutely ill. She had a high fever, a very low blood pressure, and a generalized rash that was, in all probability, a drug reaction to her previous antibiotics.

The Schnells readily agreed to my suggestion that she be immediately transferred to St. Joseph's Hospital in Milwaukee. There and at Milwaukee County General Hospital, I had been studying combinations of the newer antibiotics in endocarditis by the tube dilution method. Based on this experience, I started Diane on the combination of Lincomycin and Gentamycin. The tube dilation studies confirmed that this was the combination of antibiotics that might be of help. She made a rapid clinical response to 4 grams of Lincomycin and 500 mg of Gentamycin given in combination intravenously. These were continued for 4 weeks and blood cultures became negative and she became afebrile. During this time, I got to know Diane as an optimistic teenager who went along cheerfully with the difficulties of prolonged intravenous antibiotic therapy that were present in 1962. I also got to know her parents who were the quintessential examples of dedicated parents. They stood by Diane for the rest of their lives.

CHAPTER THREE – Second and Third Bouts of Bacterial Endocarditis – Streptococcal Viridians and Penicillin Resistant Staphylococcal

Diane returned from Milwaukee to Waukesha in December of 1962 and resumed a normal life. Diane's father's brewery business was sold in Waukesha and in 1964 he moved his family to Woodbury, New York to run a bakery that he and his partners had purchased.

Several months after they arrived, Diane began to run a fever and gallstones were found. Because of this, her gall bladder was removed on August 24, 1964 at Syosset Hospital in Stoneybrook, New York. She became feverish after the operation. Blood cultures revealed streptococcal viridians, the most common type of bacteria that causes bacterial endocarditis. The resident physician did not consider subacute bacterial endocarditis as the cause of her fever and treated her empirically with Novobiocyn and Tetracycline. Her fever abated and she was discharged. This information I obtained from her hospital record, which was provided by the Syosset Hospital. Several weeks after discharge, she developed a high fever and was admitted to the New York Medical School Hospital in Manhattan. There by coincidence she came under the care of a Dr. Anderson who happened to be the wife of Dr. Harold W. Anderson, the surgeon who had taken out Diane's gall bladder at Syosset Hospital.

The doctors Anderson are still active. He is a surgeon with business interests and she is a practicing internist in the City of New York. I contacted both of them in the fall of 2008. Dr. Anderson vaguely remembered taking out Diane's gall bladder and that she had turned up several weeks later under the care of his wife who was a senior medical resident at New York Medical School University Hospital. Dr. Anderson's wife remembered Diane as a lovely, cooperative young woman. She remembered that she had been admitted to her service at the New York University Hospital and was found to have acute penicillin resistant staphylococcal bacterial endocarditis. She also remembered that Diane had not been responding to treatment with any available antibiotics and that one of the consulting infectious disease doctors knew of a new antibiotic that might be of help. I assume that the antibiotic was Lincomycin, the drug I had treated her with during her first bout of endocarditis. The consultant called the medical director of UpJohn, the pharmaceutical company that made Lincomycin and he agreed to ship a supply to New York by air. Diane's father met the plane when it landed and hand delivered the Lincomycin to Dr. Anderson. There was almost an immediate response and after a prolonged course of intravenous therapy, Diane was discharged from the hospital with negative blood cultures. Dr. Anderson did not remember any details of the treatment and a prolonged search by the record department of the hospital failed to turn up the record. A long search by a helpful employee at UpJohn also failed to yield a record of the incident that Dr. Anderson mentioned. A possibility exists that Ristocetin from the Abbott Laboratories was the antibiotic involved but Abbot's pharmacology archive department also could not find any record of what has been described.

In 1965, however, medical directors of pharmaceutical companies were scrambling to establish the efficacy of new antibiotics. As a matter of fact, I had studied Ristocetin and Lincomycin for endocarditis and either drug might have been what was used.

Be that as it may, I cannot help but believe that Dr. Anderson's remembrance of the incident must be true particularly because of the fact that she remembered that Diane's father met the plane as it landed and rushed the antibiotic to the hospital. Furthermore, in the hectic days of 1964, uses of drugs in the way that is described would have been possible.

OPERATIVE REPORT

Dr. Harold W. Anderson

September 26, 1974

*All operative reports may be skipped by the lay reader but they may be of interest to the medically trained reader.

Burton A. Waisbren, Sr.,M.D., FACP

UNIVERSITY HOSPITAL – FINAL SUMMARY

SCHNELL, DIANE
Admitted: 9/2/64
89274
Discharged: 9/26/64
Dr. Anderson

PRESENT ILLNESS.   This is a 19 year old female with the history
of having had a Pott's procedure for Tetralogy of Fallot, as an infant.
She is now admitted with the diagnosis of cholelithiasis. Patient had
intermittent right upper quadrant pain, associated with nausea and
some vomiting, brought on by fried food. GB series prior to admission
demonstrated cholelithiasis. Patient was also known to have jaundice
prior to admission.

PHYSICAL EXAMINATION.   A normal white female in no acute
distress. She did not appear acutely ill. Thrill palpable over the apex,
and the PMI is at the 5th ICS 1 cm lateral to the MCL. A harsh systolic
murmur at the apex is noted.

HOSPITAL COURSE.   The patient was operated on 9/4/64, where
a cholecystectomy and common duct exploration with insertion of
a T-tube was carried out. Postoperatively the patient drained very
little, and the drain was pulled 2 days postoperatively. Following this
the patient began to spike temperatures ranging from 103 to 102.
Patient was placed on antibiotic therapy consisting of tetracycline and
eventually Novobiocin. With continuation of spiking temperatures
the possibility of subhepatic abscess was considered, but no evidence
was ever found. The patient improved slowly, continuing to spike
fevers occasionally, eventually all antibiotics were discontinued after
the patient had an allergic reaction apparently to streptomycin,
manifesting itself with a temperature spike to 105 and a generalized
body eruption, maclurpapular and erythematous in nature. This
subsided spontaneously after all antibiotics discontnued. Patient was
afebrile for 3 days prior to discharge and improved symptomatically.

<u>FINAL DIAGNOSIS.</u> Cholecystitis and cholelithiasis.

Dr. Engler/rs/AMTS
   10/5/64

CHAPTER FOUR - Fourth Bout of Endocarditis Due to a Gram Positive Bacilli that was Treated at an Air Base in Colorado, 1970

While living in Woodbury, New York Diane met her first husband, Michael Pontrelli. They were married in May of 1969 in Waukesha, Wisconsin shortly after Diane's family moved back there to open a bowling alley. At the time of the wedding he was serving in the United States Air Force and they were scheduled to reside at Tinker Air Force Base in Oklahoma City, Oklahoma.

A month after Diane and her husband arrived at the Tinker Air Force Base in July of 1970. Diane again began to run a high fever. She came under the care of Captain Joseph Noble who was in charge of cardiology at the air base. He recognized the possibility of recurrent endocarditis and drew six blood cultures. They all revealed bacteria that was never positively identified. Several laboratories suggested that it was a rare form of a gram-positive bacillus.

At Diane's request, Dr. Noble called me and informed me that she had classic subacute bacterial endocarditis due to this organism. He said he had no experience with this type of organism and said that he would follow Diane's request that he seek my suggestions for management. Since Diane had tolerated Lincomycin and Gentamycin when they were used in Milwaukee, I suggested that she be given 12 grams of Lincomycin and one gram of Gentamycin intravenously daily for a month and that he send the organism to the microbiology laboratory at UpJohn Pharmacology Company in Michigan for sensitivity tests. This was done and although they could not positively identify the organism, they found it to be sensitive to Lincomycin. I had been evaluating Lincomycin for this company and they were glad to help.

Diane tolerated the course of intravenous Lincomycin and Gentamycin well and made an excellent clinical response. As was my practice, her kidney function and auditory nerves were monitored weekly and showed neither the kidney nor the auditory nerve damage that are sometimes found with Gentamycin.

Diane's husband obtained a hardship discharge from the Air Force and the couple returned home to Waukesha in later 1970.

Coincidentally, Dr. Noble had been beautifully trained under the renowned cardiologist Dr. Hurst who was head of the department and a professor at Emery Medical School. Just before entering the Air Force to serve his required stint in the service, he had participated in a symposium on congenital heart disease in Atlanta, Georgia. There he had heard Dr. John Kirklin of the Mayo Clinic who had just set up a cardiac surgery program at the University of Alabama discuss his new approach to corrective surgery for the Tetralogy of Fallot. This consisted of taking down Dr. Potts connection between the aorta and the pulmonary artery and substituting it for a connection between the right ventricle and pulmonary artery that used a pig's aorta as a conduit. Dr. Kirklin had devised the method of treatment because by the late 1960s, subacute bacterial endocarditis was a known complication of the Potts operation for the Tetralogy of Fallot.

Dr. Noble suggested to me that Diane and her family contact Dr. John Kirklin to see whether he thought she was a candidate for his new procedure. He suggested that both he and I should contact Dr. Kirklin in regard to Diane. We did this and Dr. Kirklin graciously replied that he would be glad to see Diane and her family. In January 1971 Diane and her parents went to Alabama to consult with Dr John Kirklin.

CHAPTER FIVE - Second and Third Open Heart Operations Performed by Dr. John Kirklin at the Alabama Medical School Cardiac Center 1971 and 1975

Diane and her parents met with Dr. John Kirklin in early 1971. At this meeting he discussed with them the rationale for his new approach for cardiac surgery for individuals who had had the Potts operation. The main reason for the operation was the high incidence of bacterial endocarditus in long time survivors of the Potts operation. Of course the Schnells were well aware that bacterial endocarditus occurred in Potts operation survivors.

John Kirklin's operation consisted of closing the opening between the aorta and the artery leading from the ventricle and supplanting it with Dacron conduit that contained a homograph aortic valve, which took the blood from the right ventricle to the pulmonary artery that led away from the right ventricle. This bypassed the obstructed valve of the right ventricle. He also closed the opening between the two ventricles, which allowed the deoxygenated blood to get into the left ventricle. He carefully explained the rationales for his procedure and his results to date. Diane and her parents thought it over and decided to have the procedure done.

Dr John Kirklin's team did a careful preliminary cardiac work-up and surgery was performed as explained above in April 1971.

Diane's father told me of an incident that was not included in the operative report. Two hours into the operation, Dr. John Kirklin came into the waiting room and informed the family that the pig aortic shunt that he had planned to use turned out to be a "bad fit" so he had to call the shunt's purveyor in another city for a replacement. He said that the replacement was being flown in and should arrive shortly. This delayed completion of the operation for several hours. It is interesting to note that this was the second mercy flight that helped Diane to survive. The first one occurred when a life saving antibiotic was flown in from the midwest to The New York Medical School Hospital in New York.

Aside from the above the operation went smoothly and Diane had an excellent convalescence. She returned home and was able to help out at her father's bowling alley. During the next four years I saw Diane at regular intervals and while she was not overly active she seemed to be getting along well. However, in mid 1975 there was an obvious change in her condition. She became short of breath and went into mild heart failure which was controlled by digoxin and a diuretic. Several consultations with a local cardiologist resulted in the excellent suggestion that she return for a check up with Kirklin's cardiac team in Alabama. All concerned agreed and arrangements were made for her to see Dr. John Kirklin again in Alabama. A complete evaluation was done by his cardiac team and the conclusion was reached that the shunt had ceased to function fully and should be replaced. I could not help but feel that the advice of these experts should be followed. All agreed after prolonged explanations and discussions and Dr. John Kirklin found what he expected during the operation. The conduit had become compressed and was not functioning satisfactorily. The compressed conduit was removed and a new conduit consisting of a heterograft valve external conduit was sewn in that again went from the right ventricle into the pulmonary artery in December 1975.

Shortly after the first operation by Dr Kirklin in 1971 Diane's marriage broke up and she had an amicable divorce. She had moved on with her life to the point where in addition to working at the bowling alley one night a week she took on a job as a wig saleswoman at a local department store. As happens, in late 1974, she had met a new "Mr. Wonderful" who eventually became her second husband who was devotedly by her side the rest of her life.

When Diane and her parents went down to Alabama to be evaluated by Dr. Kirklin's staff in August of 1975, they openly discussed the prospects for the couple having children after they got married. Their opinion was that with the operation that this would be possible. They turned out to be correct. Diane and Stephen Cummings were married on September 29, 1975. They had two children with uncomplicated pregnancies that resulted in births on February 2, 1977 and on June 10, 1979. Diane's devotion and care mirrored that of her quintessential mother and eventually six grand children were added to the family.

OPERATIVE REPORT

Dr. John Kirklin's First Operation

April 14, 1971

Burton A. Waisbren, Sr.,M.D., FACP

The University of Alabama in Birmingham
The Medical Center/UNIVERSITY OF ALABAMA HOSPITALS
AND CLINICS

OPERATION

<u>NAME:</u> PONTRELLI, Diane
<u>HOSP. No.:</u> E25-25-4
<u>ROOM:</u> 431
<u>SURG.:</u> Dr. J. Kirklin
<u>ASSIST:</u> Drs. Pacifico, Balch, Mr. Harvey
<u>DATE OPER. OR E.D. VISIT:</u> 4-14-71__
<u>ADMITTED:</u>
<u>DISCHARGED:</u>
<u>DOCTOR/SERV.:_</u>
<u>DICTATED:</u> 4-14-71__
<u>TRANSCRIBED:</u> 4-14-71

PREOP DIAGNOSIS: Probable double outlet, left ventricle, with functioning left Pott's anastomosis and stenosis of the left pulmonary artery.

POSTOP DIAGNOSIS: Same.

OPERATION: Closure of previously constructed Pott's anastomosis; pericardial enlargement of stenotic area of left pulmonary artery; repair of ventricular septal defect; creation of external conduit from right ventricle to pulmonary artery; temporary cardiopulmonary bypass with total circulatory arrest.

A primary median sternotomy incision was made and the left femoral artery was exposed through a vertical incision. The left saphenous vein was cannulated to provide a large central venous line. The findings were unusual, but I have examined the heart very carefully and I am quite confident of these observation. The Pott's anastomosis was about 5 x 3 mm. in size and of course was functioning. Just proximal to the anastomosis, there was a high grade stenosis of the **left pulmonary artery,** so that the orifice was no more than about **6 x 7 mm. in diameter.** The ventricular mass was large and prior to opening the ventricle, I thought that the right ventricle was as usual, markedly hypertrophied and enlarged, and that the left ventricle was perhaps slightly abnormally small for a patient with a **Pott's anastomosis.** In any event, there was a very under developed infundibulum and a main pulmonary artery that was of moderate size. The pulmonary valve and the aortic valve seemed to lye at about the same level, head, footwise, but the pulmonary valve seemed maybe slightly anterior. The aorta was rather markedly enlarged, and from its external aspect, we would have said that it was dextroposed. However, we found in fact that the right ventricle had a somewhat small cavity and into it of course, entered the tricuspid valve. There was a **large typical high ventricular septal defect,** about 12 x 10 mm. in diameter. However, the aorta was absolutely not at all dextroposed. In addition to this large defect, there was just about 5 mm. anterior to it, **another small ventricular septal defect** and low down in the muscular septum, far interiorly were three or four additional Swiss cheese types of defects. Thus, there was no great vessel coming off the right ventricle. When I inadvertently opened the left ventricle, by palpating in it, I could determine that the aorta arose clearly and completely from the left ventricle. I could not put a finger up in the infundibulum, beneath the pulmonary artery, but later opened this infundibulum and saw a small communication from it *into the left ventricle.* Thus I am confident that both great arteries, in fact emerged from the left ventricle. The mitral valve entered the left ventricle. There was obviously **extremely severe pulmonary stenosis,** which was near pulmonary atresia. There were no anomalies of pulmonary or systemic venous return. The anterior descending coronary artery came from the right coronary artery and of course was very oblique, downward into the left in its direction because of the peculiar relation of the two ventricles to each other. In the interior of the right acrium was normal to palpation.___

Burton A. Waisbren, Sr.,M.D., FACP

The University of Alabama in Birmingham
The Medical Center/UNIVERSITY OF ALABAMA HOSPITALS AND CLINICS

NAME: PONTRELLI, Diane
HOSP. No.: E25-25-45
ROOM: 431
SURG.:
ASSIST:
DATE OPER. OR E.D. VISIT:
ADMITTED:
DISCHARGED:
DOCTOR/SERV.:
DICTATED:
TRANSCRIBED:

PG. II

Cardiopulmonary bypass was established at 2.2 liters per minute per square meter for a total of 195 minutes. With digital occlusion of the Pott's anastomosis and using cardiopulmonary bypass, the patient's body temperature was reduced to 22 degrees centigrade and total circulatory arrest established for 25 minutes. During this time, we made a longitudinal incision in the left pulmonary artery and closed the Pott's anastomosis with interrupted and continuous #4-0 silk sutures. The incision in the left pulmonary artery was then extended both proximal and distal to the area of stenosis and this was repaired by suturing into place a sizable piece of pericardium. This I am confident, enlarged that stenotic area. Cardiopulmonary bypass was then re-established. We made a small incision to the left of what later proved to be the anterior descending coronary artery (although this time, we thought it was just the usual oblique artery across the right ventricular out flow tract) and explored within the left ventricle. This incision was then closed with two rows of continuous silk. We then made a transverse incision in the right ventricle, excising a button of right ventricular musculature, since I knew now we would have to use a conduit. The ventricular septal defect was then repaired by suturing into place a piece of knitted Dacron. Additional sutures were placed and I think we essentially closed all of the multiple swiss cheese types of defects. We then made a transverse incision in the infundibulum, beneath the pulmonary artery, and from here closed with interrupted sutures of the communication from left ventricle in this infundibulum. This incision was then closed and we made a longitudinal incision on the main pulmonary area. **Dr. Pacifico had meanwhile fashioned our usual composite Dacron conduit,** containing the homograft aortic valve and the distal end of this was sutured end-to-side to the opening in the pulmonary artery. The proximal end was then sutured to the aperture in the right ventricle using continuous Mersilene sutures throughout. The left ventricular vent which had been in place throughout was removed and the stab wound closed. Cardiopulmonary bypass then gradually was discontinued, decannulation effective, the right atrial appendage ligated and transfixed, the stab wound in right atrium closed with a Purse-String stitch, and the femoral artery reconstructed. In spite of the long operative procedure, the hemodynamic state was good and pulmonary artery pressure was low. **An extremely prolonged time was spent** in establishing hemostasis. Polyvinyl catheters were brought out from right and left atrium for pressure measurements, two catheters were brought out from the pericardial space. The incision was closed as usual.

Dr. John Kirklin/mw

OPERATIVE REPORT

Dr. John Kirklin's Second Operation

December 17, 1975

The University of Alabama in Birmingham
The Medical Center/UNIVERSITY OF ALABAMA HOSPITALS
AND CLINICS

NAME: Diane Schnell Cummings
HOSP. No.: E 25 25 45
ROOM:
SURG.:
ASSIST:
DATE OPER. OR E.D. VISIT:
ADMITTED: 12/7/75
DISCHARGED: 12/21/75
DOCTOR/SERV.: Dr. Kirklin-CVS_
DICTATED: 12/22/75_
TRANSCRIBED: 12/26/75

A patient of Dr. Burton Waisbren.
200 North Water
Milwaukee, Wisconsin 53202

DIAGNOSIS: Conduit compression with pumonic stenosis and pulmonic insufficiency.

Summary: This is a 30 YOWF, status post Pott's anastomosis for tetralogy of Fallot at age 18 months and status post complete repair on 4/14/71 of double outlet left ventricle (with homograft valve external conduit). Presents now with enlargement of the right ventricle and the right atrium and with recent pedal edema. The above symptoms were thought to be due to compression on the previously placed external conduit.

PROCEDURE: Replacement of valved external conduit with heterograft valved external conduit (Hancock, #P4937-22); preliminary femero-femoral bypass with induction of hyothermis; temporary cardiopulmonary bypass, 12/12/75.

FINDINGS: The conduit was found to be tightly compressed between the left side of the sternum and the ventricular mass. There seemed to be no obstruction of either the proximal or the distal anastomosis.

HOSPITAL COURSE: The postop course was satisfactory with immediate postop cardiac index of 3.08. On postop day two, she developed a Grade II/VI pulmonary dysfunction which cleared with intensive physiotherapy. She maintained a low grade temp. for which Chloromycetin was continued through postop day five. A systolic murmur continued to be heard but no S-3 or S-4 was present. Seven day studies included: Chest X-ray –left pleural effusion; EKG, sinus rhythm 100 per minute with no acute changes. Lab: Potassium 4.2, WBC 8200, hemoglobin 9.6. Outpatient appointments 12/22/75. No tests for outpatient clinic. Discharge medications: Potassiium Chloride 1 tbs. t.i.d. and Lasix 40 gm q.a.m. both to be continued for ten days and then every other day for ten days, Iron Sulfate 300 mg t.i.d. for three weeks, ½ gram sodium diet for one month.

Ed Colvins, M.D.: dw

The University of Alabama in Birmingham
The Medical Center/UNIVERSITY OF ALABAMA HOSPITALS AND CLINICS

NAME: Diane Schnell Cummings
HOSP. No.: E 25 25 45
ROOM:
SURG.:
ASSIST:
DATE OPER. OR E.D. VISIT:
ADMITTED: 12/7/75
DISCHARGED: 12/21/75
DOCTOR/SERV.: Dr. Kirklin-CVS
DICTATED: 12/22/75
TRANSCRIBED: 12/26/75

A patient of Dr. Burton Waisbren.
200 North Water
Milwaukee, Wisconsin 53202

DIAGNOSIS: Conduit compression with pumonic stenosis and pulmonic insufficiency.

Summary: This is a 30 YOWF, status post Pott's anastomosis for tetralogy of Fallot at age 18 months and status post complete repair on 4/14/71 of double outlet left ventricle (with homograft valve external conduit). Presents now with enlargement of the right ventricle and the right atrium and with recent pedal edema. The above symptoms were thought to be due to compression on the previously placed external conduit.

PROCEDURE: Replacement of valved external conduit with heterograft valved external conduit (Hancock, #P4937-22); preliminary femero-femoral bypass with induction of hyothermis; temporary cardiopulmonary bypass, 12/12/75.

FINDINGS: The conduit was found to be tightly compressed between the left side of the sternum and the ventricular mass. There seemed to be no obstruction of either the proximal or the distal anastomosis.

HOSPITAL COURSE: The postop course was satisfactory with immediate postop cardiac index of 3.08. On postop day two, she developed a Grade II/VI pulmonary dysfunction which cleared with intensive physiotherapy. She maintained a low grade temp. for which Chloromycetin was continued through postop day five. A systolic murmur continued to be heard but no S-3 or S-4 was present. Seven day studies included: Chest X-ray –left pleural effusion; EKG, sinus rhythm 100 per minute with no acute changes. Lab: Potassium 4.2, WBC 8200, hemoglobin 9.6. Outpatient appointments 12/22/75. No tests for outpatient clinic. Discharge medications: Potassiium Chloride 1 tbs. t.i.d. and Lasix 40 gm q.a.m. both to be continued for ten days and then every other day for ten days, Iron Sulfate 300 mg t.i.d. for three weeks, ½ gram sodium diet for one month.

Ed Colvins, M.D.: dw

The University of Alabama in Birmingham
The Medical Center/UNIVERSITY OF ALABAMA HOSPITALS AND CLINICS

NAME: Diane Cummings
HOSP. No.: E25-25-45_
ROOM: 242
SURG.: Dr. Kirklin
ASSIST: Dr. Parr and Mr. Silver_
DATE OPER. OR E.D. VISIT: 12/12/75
ADMITTED:
DISCHARGED:
DOCTOR/SERV.:
DICTATED: 12/12/75
TRANSCRIBED: 12/25/75

PREOPERATIVE DIAGNOSIS: Postoperative repair of double outlet left ventricle with pulmonary stenosis, with severe compression of valved external conduit between right ventricle and pulmonary artery.

POSTOPERATIVE DIAGNOSIS: Same.

OPERATION: Replacement of valved external conduit with heterograft valved external conduit (Hancock, #P4937-22); preliminary famerofemoral bypass with induction of hypothermis; temporary cardiopulmonary bypass.

Because we anticipated problems opening the sternum without getting into the valved external condit the left famoral artery and femoral vein were exposed. Both were cannulated and cardiopulmonary bypass was established for a total elapsed time of 130 mins. We were able to get very good flows, up to 2.0 with this peripheral connulation and the patient's body temperature was reduced with it to 31 degrees centigrade in about 18 mins. Then the secondary median sternotomy incision was made. *The conduit was found to be tightly compressed between the left side of the sternum and the ventricular mass.* There seemed to be no obstruction at either the proximal or distal anastomosis.

After splitting the sternum, we mobilized the conduit away from the undersurface of the sternum. We mobilized just enough of the heart to allow us to place two purse-string sutures in the right atrium. Cardiopulmonary bypass was then interrupted for two minutes while we placed two #6 venous cannulse through these purse string sutures and established total cardiopulmonary bypass in this way. Because of the dense scarring, we did not dissect out the cavaae and sis not use caval tapes. The perfusion was at 2.0 liters per min. per square meter and at 28 degrees centigrade. We completely dissected out the conduit and removed it from its attachment to the pulmonary artery distally and the right ventricle proximally. Before heparinizing the patient, we had preclotted a 22 mm *Hancock heterograft conduit.* This was then trimmed appropriately so as to make a reversed C shape. The distal anastomosis was then made with continuous 4-0 Prolene suture. The proximal anastomosis was similarly made by our usual technique. The patient was then rewarmed, cardiopulmonary bypass discontinued, decannulation effected, the stab wounds in right atrium closed with purse string sutures, and the left femoral artery and vein reconstructed. The memodynamic state was good. Peak pressure in the cavity of the right ventricle was 25 while the systemic arterial pressure was 95. A prolonged period of time was spent in establishing hemostasis. Polyvinyl catheters were brought out from right atrium for pressure measurements postoperatively. Two catheters were brought out from the pericardial space and one from the left pleural space. Two right atrial and a right ventricular myocardial wires were left as precautions, the incision was closed as usual.

John W. Kirklin, M.D./cow

DISCHARGE SUMMARY

NAME: Cummings, Diane J.   MED.REC.NO.: 0446103

PHYSICAL EXAMINATION: Examination was significant for a III/VI systolic murmur, IV/VI systolic murmur over the pulmonic area, increased jugular venous distentions, and clear lung fields. The patient also had shifting abdominal dullness, consistent with ascites and trace pedal edema bilaterally.

HOSPITAL COURSE: The patient was taken to the operating room on 1/19/93 for removal of an obstructed valve extracardiac conduit and placement of a 21 mm aortic homograft extracardiac conduit. The patient tolerated the procedure well and was taken to the CICU in stable condition. She was extubated late on postoperative day number one and was weaned off of pressors and transferred to the floor on postoperative day number three. On postoperative day number one, the patient reverted to atrial fibrillation and was started on digoxin as per the Arrhythmia Service. She was kept on her atrial pacer while on the floor, but this was eventually discontinued. When it was discontinued the patient went into atrial flutter and went into atrial fibrillation and spontaneously into junctional rhythm, and kept on alternating rhythms, and finally patient spontaneously converted to sinus. When the patient was initially transferred to the floor she initially complained of nausea and vomiting, and no evidence of orthostasis was obtained. The patient's digoxin level at this point was 1.2. Because of the persistent alternating rhythms, we kept the patient on her dose of digoxin. The Arrhythmia Service, however, recommended that the digoxin be discontinued secondary to possible digitoxin toxicity. The recommendations were followed, and the digoxin was discontinued, and the patient's rhythm fluctuations seemed to have slowed down and stayed more in sinus. Of interest, the patient's nausea and vomiting improved prior to the discontinuation of the digoxin. The patient continued to progress well. She was increasing her p.o. intake and was beginning to ambulate independently. Two days prior to her discharge, the patient had an isolated 13 beat run of supraventricular tachycardia. This spontaneously resolved with no further arrhythmias. The patient was in sinus rhythm at the time of discharge.

The patient's postoperative studies were as follows: Echocardiogram revealed no pericardial effusion, right loculated pleural effusion, and trivial atrial insufficiency. The patient also had no residual VSD and a good left ventricular function with an EF of 55-60%. The conduit was functioning well, and the maximum velocity across the homograft was 2.5 M/sec. with a right ventricular systolic pressure of 35-40 mmHg. Chest X-ray revealed cardiomegaly, right pleural effusion, small left pleural effusion, and possible small pericardial effusion. Overall, this was a satisfactory postoperative chest. The patient's EKG revealed sinus tachycardia with a right bundle branch block and some Q-waves in the inferior leads and the lateral precordial leads. Her fluid balance profile showed sodium of 138, potassium 3.3 chloride 98, bicard 24, glucose 87m Bun 17, creatinine 1.0, SGOT 70, total bilirubin 3.4, direct billi 2.3. The patient's preoperative values were SGOT 28, total bilirubin of 2.7, direct bili of 0.7. These postoperative values are elevated, but are stable. The patient's CBC revealed WBC of 9.5, hemoglobin 10.6, hematocrit 30, platolots 158.

CHAPTER SIX – Fourth open heart operation performed by Dr. James Kirklin 1993 and a moment of truth

Between 1975 and 1992 Diane and Stephen had an "Ozzie & Harriet" (from the television series) type of relationship. The children were active and darling and Diane was involved, caring, and physically functioning almost normally although I think she probably was pushing herself a bit. I saw her on visits at monthly or two monthly intervals and was involved with her obstetricians during her pregnancies, which went smoothly.

In early 1992 things began to change. Although she never complained she became short of breath and had significant swelling at her lower extremities. I felt she was in mild heart failure and this responded to digoxin, a diuretic and salt restrictions.

I felt that a preemptive examination by Dr. John Kirklin was in order and I wrote to him for an appointment. I was informed that he had recently retired and that his son, Dr. James Kirklin had taken over his duties. I wrote to Dr. James Kirklin who with his father's courtly manner agreed to see her in follow-up. Diane and her husband agreed to see Dr. James Kirklin in Alabama in December 1992. He had assumed the leadership of the cardiac surgery department at the University of Alabama and had an impressive team in place. After an exhaustive evaluation, which included a heart catheterization, they concluded that the second conduit had clotted off and it should be replaced. When Diane got back I called her in to discuss the matter with her.

During this office visit a "moment of truth" occurred between us that I never will forget. When I broached to her that in my opinion she needed another open-heart operation, this quiet, accepting, gentle woman, who at the time was 51 years old, seemed to suddenly take the part of her strong determined mother who I knew not only as Diane's mother but as a patient. She jutted out her jaw, looked me straight in the eye and said, "Dr. Waisbren since I was a little girl I have known that I have had a serious health problem and even then I was determined to accept it and live an active full life. I have followed your suggestions, which have worked out since I first saw you forty years ago and I want to continue to do so. What do you suggest I do?" I was taken aback but pulled myself together and said, "Diane I think you should do what Dr. Kirklin says." "That settles it", she said, "make the arrangements." This "moment of truth" between us stayed with me and gave me the courage to orchestrate what we did over the next 15 years. Neither of us mentioned this conversation again.

Dr. James Kirklin did the fourth open-heart operation in January of 1993. He replaced the shunt that his father had put in, in 1975. His operative report follows at the end of this chapter.

Diane recovered well from the operation from which there were no complications. As discussed by her husband in Chapter Nine, she led an active life as a mother, wife and then a grandmother.

I continued to see her in monitoring office calls and until 2001 things went comparatively smoothly. She intermittently had mild heart failure, which responded to diuretics and salt restriction. Monitoring her lipids, kidney and liver function revealed normal values. She began to have auricular fibrillation for which I placed her on Coumadin (an anticoagulant). I repeatedly told her that she was trying to do too much but aside from that not much was happening.

OPERATIVE REPORT

Dr. James Kirklin's Operation

January 1, 1993

Burton A. Waisbren, Sr., M.D., FACP

The University of Alabama in Birmingham
The Medical Center/UNIVERSITY OF ALABAMA HOSPITALS AND CLINICS

OPERATION NOTE page 1

<u>NAME</u>: CUMINGS, DIANE J.
<u>MED.REC.NO.</u>: 0446103
<u>ROOM</u>:
<u>SURG</u>: DR. JAMES K. KIRKLIN
<u>ASSIST</u>: DR. TREY PLUSCHT/DR.MITCH WILCUTT
<u>SURG. SIGN.</u>:
<u>DATE OPER.</u>: 01/19/93
<u>ADMITTED</u>:
<u>DISCHARGED</u>:
<u>SERVICE</u>: DR. JAMES K. KIRKLIN
<u>DICTATED</u>: 01/19/93
<u>TRANSCRIBED</u>: 01/19/93
<u>DOTO/SERV. SIGN.</u>:

PREOPERATIVE DIAGNOSIS: Status post repair of double inlet, left ventricle, ventricular septal defect, severe pulmonary stenosis. Staus post placement of right ventricular to pulmonary artery valve extracardiac conduit, status post replacement of that conduit with a porcine valve extracardiac conduit (17 years ago), severe conduit obstruction with right ventricular failure and ascites.

POSTOPERATIVE DIAGNOSIS: Same.

OPERATION: Removal obstructed valve extracardiac conduit; placement

- 36 -

of a 21 mm aortic homograft valve
extracardiac conduit (2192066),
temporary cardiopulmonary
bypass, mild hypothermia.

INDICATIONS FOR OPERATION: This delightful 48 year old
woman had previously undergone repair of tetralogy of double outlet
left ventricle and pulmonary stenosis by Dr. John Kirklin. The left
femoral artery and vein were cannulated after heparinizing the patient.
A median sternotomy was then made. The conduit was densely
adherent to the ribs on the left side and was obviously compressed
and stenotic. Within the conduit, there was a thick new intimal peel.
In addition, the valve itself was severely degenerated. We could not
effectively assess the size of the ventricular chambers because we only
dissected out enough to allow exposure of the conduit.

Cardiopulmonary bypass was established at 2.2 liters/min./meter sq.
for 115 min. The conduit was entered and then complete excised
except for a thin rim of Dacron graft at each end. The new intimal peel
was entirely removed and there was good access into the pulmonary
artery, as well as the right ventricle.

A 21 mm aortic homograft had been prepared, it was trimmed just
distal to the commissures. The distal anastomosis was constructed
with continuous 4-0 Prolene. Proximally, it was anastomosed to
the proximal portion of the right ventriculotomy. The remainder
of the right ventriculotomy was closed with a small hood of bovine
pericardium. Upon completion, it looked very nice.

The University of Alabama in Birmingham
The Medical Center/UNIVERSITY OF ALABAMA HOSPITALS
AND CLINICS

DISCHARGE SUMMARY

NAME: CUMMINGS, DIANE J.
MED.REC.NO. : 0446103
ROOM:
SERVICE: DR. JAMES K. KIRKLIN/1327
ADMITTED: 01/13/93
DISCHARGED: 01/29/93
DICTATED: 01/29/93
TRANSCRIBED: 02/09/93

PRIMARY DIAGNOSIS: Right heart failure, secondary to obstructed extracardiac conduit.

OTHER DIAGNOSES: Patient has a history of tricuspid atresia, double outlet left ventricle, status post multiple surgical repairs.

PRINCIPLE PROCEDURE: Removal of obstructed valve, extracardiac conduit and placement of a 21 mm aortic homograft extracardiac conduit.

HISTORY OF PRESENT ILLNESS: The patient is a 48 year old white female with a congenital heart anomaly which was a double outlet left ventricle, status post multiple surgical repairs. The patient had been doing well until October 1992, when she developed shortness of breath, lower extremity edema, and ascites. The patient was admitted to Dr. Sharon Dailey's service in right heart failure. An MRI of the heart revealed right atrial enlargement, patent conduit, and had a heterograft that was neither incomopetent nor stenotic.

Cardiac catheterization revealed and obstructed heterograft with a right ventricular systolic pressure of about 100 and a mean right atrial pressure of 25. The catheterization also revealed a moderate tricuspid regurgitation, and the right atrial enlargement. Also, a grade II aortic insufficiency, stenosis of the left ventricular outflow tract, and good right ventricular systolic function were also noted. A 2-D echo and color Doppler confirmed the above findings; and the echo also noted a large right pleural effusion.

PAST MEDICAL HISTORY: The patient is status post repair of a double outlet left ventricle, status post repair of a VSD, and status post repair of severe pulmonary artery stenosis. The patient is also status post a Pott's shunt at age 18 months; status post closure of Potts and closure of multiple VSDs (already mentioned). There 1971, and a right ventricular-to-PA heterograft conduit in 1975. Patient has also had three episodes of sub acute bacterial endocarditis (Staph, aureus, Strep. Viridians, Lactobacillus).

CURRENT MEDICATIONS: (1) Minipres 1 mg q.a.m. and q.p.m.; (2) digoxin 0.25 mg p.o. q.d.; (3) Cipro 500 mg p.o. b.i.d.; (4) Lasix 40 mg p.o. b.i.d.; (5) K-Kur 10 mg p.o. b.i.d.

ALLERGIES: Patient is allergic to penicillin, Keflex, erythromycin, streptomycin, and oxacillin.

CHAPTER SEVEN -Events leading up to her fifth open heart procedure

In early 2000 things began to change. When she walked into the office she had lost the spring in her step. She looked worn out. Her edema became worse and it was obvious that things were not going well. Consultations with several cardiologist in Milwaukee did not lead to any helpful suggestions.

I prevailed with her to have a preemptive visit with Dr. James Kirklin. His team went over her and concluded that all possible was being done for her and that further surgery was not indicated. Things worsened with her edema to the extent that she spent much of her day on the living room couch with her legs propped up with pillows. She tried to put up on an optimistic face but she was obviously depressed.

At that point I felt that a cardiac transplant should be considered. She and her husband agreed that this should be considered on a quality of life basis. St Luke's Medical Center in Milwaukee had developed a fine heart transplant service so they were consulted. Dr. Couch, the director of that service, after an examination accepted her for heart transplant and she was put on a waiting list. They assumed cardiac management while she was waiting to be called. This management through St Luke's transplant team brought some measured improvement and Diane's spirits rose. However, after six months on the waiting list, due to insurance change, we found that Diane would have to be referred to one of the new insurers' preferred hospitals for transplantation treatment to be fully covered.

Accordingly, I referred her to the University of Wisconsin Madison Medical Heart Failure and Heart Transplant Service. After another exhaustive work up the cardiologists in charge suggested that she be seen by Dr. Dearani of the Mayo Clinic who was pioneering reconstruction of the right ventricular heart valve whose obstruction was the main cause of the Tetralogy of Falot. All concerned felt that this was a good suggestion and arrangements were made for Diane to see Dr. Dearani. After another exhaustive work up Dr. Dearani and his cardiac team accepted Diane as a candidate for a plastic repair of her bicuspid valve (the valve at the outlet of the right ventricle). Dr. Dearani operated upon Diane on December 1, 2003. While his operative report, which follows this chapter, makes it look easy one can only imagine the skill and courage that was exhibited in the operation that removed the shunt which seemed to be functioning and repaired the tricuspid valve which when he got done was functioning well. This was done in an operative field that had been visited four previous times.

Postoperatively, from a cardiac standpoint all went well but unfortunately her kidneys failed completely so she had to be put on dialysis which continued until her death in January, 2007, three years later. The dialysis was done at a center at Waukesha Memorial Hospital. She accepted the dialysis with her usual good cheer.

OPERATIVE REPORT

Dr. Dearani's Operation

December 1, 2003

Burton A. Waisbren, Sr.,M.D., FACP

CURRENT OPERATIVE REPORT CONT.   Page 2
MAYO CLINIC
6-148-982
Cummings, Mrs. Diane Jane
12/01/2003
5

Cardioplegic arrest (blood).
Intraoperative transesophageal echocardiography.

Drainage: 2 mediastinal chest tubes,
Chest tubes in both pleural spaces

OPERATIVE PROCEDURE: The patient was brought to the operating room, and monitoring lines were placed. After the usual prep and drape, a fourth-time redo sternotomy was performed without any misadventures. The aorta was closely adherent to the sternum but was dissected off without any injury. There were massive adhesions between the lung and the heart, the lung and the chest wall, and the conduit and the chest wall. A fair amount of time was spent prior to by pass with sharp and cautery dissection. We eventually gained exposure of the superior and inferior venae cavae, the right atrium, and the ascending aorta. I could not safely expose any more of the conduit without decompression of the cardiac chambers.

Heparin was administered. The ascending aorta was cannulated with a 20 French DLP cannula. The superior and inferior venae cavae were cannulated separately with right-angle venous cannulae. Caval tapes were placed. Cardiopulmonary bypass was commenced at 2.4 L/min per m2 for 132 minutes, and the perfusate was cooled to 32 degrees centigrade. The obstructed homograft conduit was then dissected off the chest wall, and the significant adhesions between the lung and the heart and the lung and the chest wall were also taken down. We eventually gained exposure of the conduit. An aortic tack vent was placed on aspiration. The aorta was occluded, and 800 cc of cold blood cardioplegia was infused in the aortic root, obtaining satisfactory asystolic arrest. Additional cardioplegia was given at 20-minute intervals during the cross-clamp period. Caval tapes were snared. An oblique right atriotomy was performed. The coronary sinus was easily visualized, and the orifice of the 6- x 10-cm right atrial diverticulum located along the inferior aspect of the ventricle was identified. The orifice was approximately 4 cm in length and was closed in two layers with running Prolene suture. This obliterated this space nicely. The mechanism of the tricuspid regurgitation was from a defect in the septal leaflet related to the ventricular septal defect patch. The tricuspid valve repair was performed by approximating the medial edge of the anterior leaflet to the medial edge of the septal leaflet with a mattress suture of Prolene backed with a felt pledget. A small transverse aortotomy was made. Inspection of the aortic valve demonstrated the nodules of Arantius to be thickened on all three cusps. The fibroelastoma was on the ventricular aspect of the noncoronary cusp and was excised without difficulty. There were no other abnormalities

SAUS MO15126
CONTINUED ON NEXT PAGE
Printed 03/28/2007 14:53

Burton A. Waisbren, Sr.,M.D., FACP

CURRENT OPERATIVE REPORT CONT.   Page 3
MAYO CLINIC
6-148-982
Cummings, Mrs. Diane Jane
12/01/2003
5

With the aortic valve. The aortotomy was closed with running 4-0 Prolene suture in two layers.

The cross-clamp was released after 23 minutes with suction on the aortic root vent. Normal sinus rhythm resumed after a single countershock. Attention was then turned to the right ventricular outflow tract. The conduit was heavily calcified and was incised longitudinally up to the pulmonary artery confluence. There had been previously placed Dacron on both the distal aspect of the reconstruction and the proximal aspect of the reconstruction. The lateral edges of the calcified homograft were endarterectomized. A piece of glutaraldehyde-preserved bovine pericardium was then sutured to close and enlarge the distal portion of the main pulmonary artery reconstruction. The right pulmonary artery accepted a 20-mm Bakes dilator and the left Horizontal mattress sutures of 2-0 Ethibond backed with felt pledgets were placed in the native pulmonary annulus with pledgets on the pulmonary artery side. A 29-mm porcine bioprosthesis was then seated without difficulty. The glutaraldehyde-preserved bovine pericardium was then sutured to the anterior sewing ring of the valve and then finally used to close the residual ventriculotomy. The conduit reconstruction lay nicely. The patient was rewarmed to 37 degrees centigrade. The right atriotomy was closed with a running 3-0 Prolene suture in two layers. Caval tapes were released prior to completing the suture line to evacuate all air from the right heart. Cardiopulmonary bypass was gradually discontinued with satisfactory hemodynamics on low-dose epinephrine, renal dose dopamine, and Nipride. Post-cardiopulmonary bypass trasesophageal echo demonstrated ventricular function to be in the low-normal range. There was trivial residual tricuspid regurgitation. The pulmonary bioprosthesis was well seated and functioning normally. There was good flow into both pulmonary arteries. There were no residual abnormalities with the aortic valve. There was mild mitral regurgitation. There was no evidence of blood flow into the residual diverticulum of the right atrium. Decannulation was accomplished and surgical sites oversewn with Prolene suture. Protamine was administered. Hemostasis was achieved. Pressures were measured, and the right ventricular pressure was 35/2 mmHg with a systemic blood pressure of 100/62 mmHg. Temporary pacing wireswere left on the free walls of the right ventricle. There were multiple air leaks in both lungs, more so on the left side. A fair amount of time was spent obtaining hemostasis and trying to control these air leaks. Flo-Seal was placed on the raw surface of the lung. We eventually gained what I felt was satisfactory hemostasis and control of the air leaks. Chest tubes were led into both pleural spaces and two in the mediastinum. The mediastinum and pleural spaces were irrigated with warm antibiotic solution. The sternum was closed with interrupted wire in the usual manner and the wound closed in layers with Vicryl.

SAUS MO15126
CONTINUED ON NEXT PAGE
Printed 03/28/2007 14:53

CURRENT OPERATIVE REPORT CONT.   Page 4
MAYO CLINIC
6-148-982
Cummings, Mrs. Diane Jane
12/01/2003
5

Intraoperative autotransfusion present.

A total of 500 cc of packed cells, 450 cc of washed cells, 500 cc of albumin, 3500 cc of Plasma-Lyte, 10 cc of heparin, 100 cc of sodium bicarbonate, and 150 cc of mannitol was used inn the Capiox-Terumo SX25 membraine oxygenatory.

A hemoconcentrator was used – 300cc removed.

    Wound Type: TYPE I – CLEAN
    Transcriptionist: lrb

CHAPTER EIGHT - The Final Course

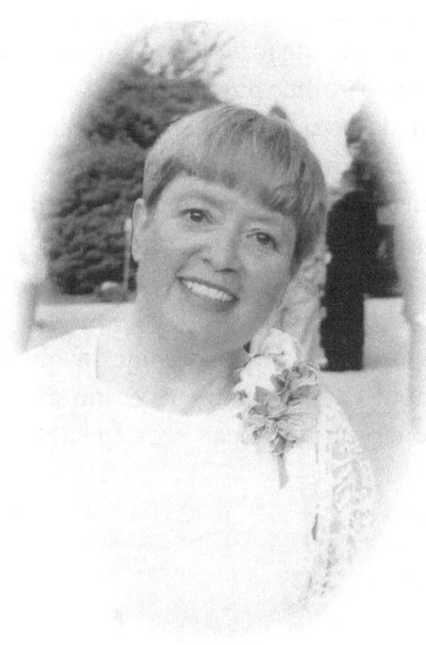

Diane with her usual good cheer tolerated biweekly dialysis for three years without complications or complaints. Her cardiac function remained satisfactory until later 2006 when I began once again to have difficulty in controlling her relatively mild heart failure. However,even with the constraints of bi-weekly dialysis, she was able to run a busy household, and to dote on her family which now included four grandchildren.

Disaster occurred on December 15, 2006. She called her husband who was at work with the news that her heart was beating very rapidly and that she couldn't breathe. He returned home and rushed her to the emergency room at Waukesha Memorial Hospital. She arrived there with ventricular tachychardia and carcinogenic shock. Under the care of the medical team at Waukesha Memorial lead by Dr. Terry Zarling, Diane made modest progress to the point where she was able to ambulate around the nurse station with oxygen. Family and close friends were encouraged that Diane's spirit would once again prevail despite her dire condition.

Dr. Zarling consulted with Dr. Michael Earing, a Mayo Clinic trained cardiologist at Children's Hospital in Milwaukee. He took interest and arranged to have Diane transferred to Froedtert Hospital in Milwaukee. However, before Diane could be transferred she experienced an incident of internal bleeding. Notwithstanding this setback, as soon as Diane was stabilized she was transferred to the cardiac intensive care unit at the Froedtert Hospital where despite valiant efforts, she could not maintain a sustainable blood pressure without large dosages of vasopressors. This was in spite of the fact that the ventricular fibrillations had been converted to auricular fibrillations.

Intractable bleeding and heart failure were too much for Diane. She continued to be unable to sustain an adequate blood pressure in spite of all efforts. She communicated to her physicians and family that she had "had enough" and wanted to peacefully die. Her husband, her family and end of life experts at Froedtert carefully considered her request and came to the conclusion that it was a reasonable one that should be granted. During the morning hours, she visited with her family and friends and at noon on January 21, 2007, the vasopressors were stopped and she quietly died.

Not to my credit I could not bring myself to become involved in her final illness that I knew would end as it did. A postmortem revealed that Dr. Dearani's pulmonary artery repair was apparently functioning.

CHAPTER NINE – Description of Diane written by Stephen Cummings, her husband

Diane could be described as a sweet, gentle, mild spoken person who was concerned about others almost to a fault. This disposition came about no doubt through her frail beginnings. Her Dr. Potts surgery was no more than a temporary fix that doctors expected would allow her to live only into her early twenties. Before the advancements that led to her later surgeries, she would have to take measured steps while others her age were running. This early start gave her awareness and appreciation of others in need. I found that she would always take time to talk and to help out.

I became aware of this concern for others when I first met Diane. She was a wig salesperson working at Chapman's, a local department store. The time had just gone by when wigs were passé in fashion. Most customers now seeking wigs were losing hair due to illness, old age and chemotherapy. She would talk to me about her customers and their problems. She no doubt kept her job because of her compassionate nature with these clients.

Her awareness could be seen in the attention that she gave to others. She seemed to take pleasure in helping out when she could. This last Christmas, while she was lying up in the hospital in critical condition, she had me running around lending our roaster to a friend that she had made in dialysis for this friend's Christmas turkey. Even in her last days she was thinking about how she could help others.

Her compassionate nature extended to animals. We had our dogs, Sparky and Muffy, tropical fish, parakeets and our cat, Midnight. In Diane's care, Muffy and Midnight were the last of their litters to pass away, living long after their brothers and sisters. Outside we had birds of all descriptions, chipmunks, mice, squirrels, fox, hawks, possum, rabbits, ground hogs and other critters, too many to mention that benefited from Diane's generous feeding. If a bird got hurt, she would take it to the Humane Society. Diane watched out for them all.

I frequently observed Diane's patient and loving manner with children. She seemed to know how to treat them whatever their stage of development. This caring nature was evident throughout our life together. She had a special place in her heart for toddlers in her Sunday school class. The neighborhood kids could always count on a free peanut butter sandwich at Diane's.

For all her care for others, I appreciate most the care that Diane had for her own family. Diane pretty much ran our family, as my job had always included a fair amount of travel. Except for outside work, I was left pretty much off the hook. I was there for the fun things, the going out to eat once a week, the taking the kids to their games, even coaching their teams on occasion, and going on vacation. But the activities that really make a family go were Diane's responsibility. The paying of the bills, the kids' homework, the planning for birthdays and Christmas, the wash and cleaning were Diane's duties. She cared for us in the same manner that she cared for everyone else. We were truly lucky.

INTRODUCTION TO APPENDIX

In this Appendix information will be presented culled from the seven volume medical record in my office that was compiled during the forty-five years that I was her primary physician. Brief paragraphs regarding the physicians that became involved in Diane's saga will be of interest to some readers. In addition readers may find the voluminous correspondence occasioned by this saga of interest. I think it illustrates the empathy and dedication of the wide variety of physicians who were involved in her care.

The references that are included will be of interest to those who want to study the evolution of treatment during the first half of the twentieth century of both congenital heart disease and bacterial endocarditis.

Finally, Dr. Martin Werra, Diane's general practitioner in Waukesha, remained deeply involved in her care until his death in 1979. He deserves mention because he represents the finest in regard to dedication to the medical profession.

THE PLAYERS

This section introduces the four surgeons who were involved in Diane's saga. Mention will also be made of the wide diversity in the United States that allowed the saga to take place. As a born and bred Midwesterner, I am proud to say that three of the four surgeons involved were born and bred in the Midwest. Dr. Potts was born and raised in Sheboygan, Wisconsin and the Kirklins were raised in Indiana and Rochester, Minnesota.

DR. POTTS

Dr. Potts was born in Sheboygan, Wisconsin, graduated Rush Medical College in Chicago. On his release from his army service in 1942, he joined the faculty of Northwestern University Medical School and rapidly rose to the position of the head cardiac surgeon at the Children's Memorial Hospital in Chicago. There he became one of the pioneers of pediatric cardiac surgery after he developed his famous operation for the Tetrology of Fallot. He operated on hundreds of patients with this disease after he did the first operation of this type on Diane. He died in 1968 at the age of 73. He had retired and moved to Florida in 1966. His last contact with Diane's parents was in 1964. They had informed him of Diane's gall bladder operation of 1964. In his letter, he suggested that they consider him making arrangements for Diane to have her defective pulmonary artery valve repaired by open heart surgery. I found this letter in Diane's seven-volume chart in my office but I have no recollection of Diane sharing it with me. Through a retrospect scope, one wonders what would have happened if the Schnells had followed through on Dr Potts' opinion regarding an operation to repair her pulmonary artery valve in 1964.

THE KIRKLINS

John Kirklin was born in Muncie, Indiana in 1917 and he died in 2004. His father became a venerated and innovative radiologist at the Mayo Clinic in Rochester, Minnesota where John was raised. He graduated Harvard University Medical School and returned to the Mayo Clinic where he was instrumental in the development of the heart lung machine that is now used universally in open heart surgery. He retired from the Mayo Clinic at age 62 and accepted an offer to form a cardiac service at the University of Alabama Medical School. There he continued his pioneering work and developed the operation that bypassed the blocked pulmonary artery valve with a shunt with porcine valve. He described this operation at a meeting in Atlanta in 1970. Dr. Joseph Noble heard his presentation and that is how Diane came to be referred to him for the operation. Dr. Kirklin did the second and third open heart operations on Diane.

Dr. James Kirklin, the son of Dr. John Kirklin, was born and raised in Rochester, Minnesota and received his medical education as did his father at Harvard University Medical School. He became a pediatric cardiac surgeon and his early achievements caused him to be selected to succeed his father as the director of the cardiac surgery program at the University of Alabama in Birmingham. Dr. James Kirklin did the fourth cardiac operation on Diane but passed on the opportunity to do further surgery in 2000.

DR. JOSEPH DEARANI

Dr. Dearani is a successor to the Kirklins at the Mayo Clinic and has already distinguished himself as a leader of correction of congenital heart defects in children.

THE DOCTORS ANDERSON

The Doctors Anderson, the surgeon and internist who took care of Diane during her illness in New York, went on to distinguished careers in their specialties. They are both still active and shared with me this recollection of how they remembered Diane's illness in New York.

DR. JOSEPH NOBLE

Dr. Joseph Noble, who had the courage to treat Diane in Colorado (with my telephone guidance), has gone on to become a beloved and active cardiologist in Indianapolis.

As I went over Diane's seven volume chart, it became apparent that the cardiologists and internists that became involved in and helped Diane during her medical saga were too many to mention in detail. As a whole, they illustrate the breadth and dedication of the medical system that has developed in this country.

The transportation system also must be mentioned as well since Diane at one time or another was treated in Chicago, New York, Birmingham, Colorado, Milwaukee, and Waukesha.

The two airplane flights that saved Diane's life, one to New York to deliver the life saving antibiotics and the other to Alabama to deliver the graft during Diane's second open heart procedure, are also worthy to mention.

The hospitals concerned were the Children's Hospital in Chicago, the hospital in Stonybrook, New York, the New York University Medical School in Manhattan, St. Joseph's, St. Luke's and Froedtert hospitals in Milwaukee, and Waukesha Memorial Hospital in Waukesha.

There were literally dozens of cardiologists who lent a hand. They include the cardiologists who were members of the teams of Dr. Potts the Kirklins, and Dr. Dearami and at St. Luke's Transplant Center, and the University of Wisconsin Cardiac Center. The physicians who were involved with the cases of endocarditis that I was not actively present at were the husband and wife surgical and internist team of the Drs. Anderson and Dr. Joseph Noble. The Andersons are still going strong and Dr. Noble is a respected, busy cardiologist in Indianapolis. They all fondly remember Diane and were glad to share with me their remembrances.

I used over the years of my association with Diane the expertise of practicing cardiologists in the Milwaukee area. Notable among them were my son, Dr. Burton Waisbren, Jr., Dr. Theodore Silver, and Dr. Rob Roth. Diane's obstetricians of course were of help in handling her deliveries.

The cooperation of Diane's insurance carrier, Blue Cross of Wisconsin, must also be mentioned. During all the years of the saga, I did not hear a "peep" from her carrier which in this day and age seems almost miraculous.

As I look back over the 45 years since Dr. Joseph Noble and I treated Diane at Tinker Air Force Base Hospital, I realize that now, in 2010, that neither I nor Dr. Noble would be able to do what we did in 1962. Not only that but now we probably would not have the courage to do it even though we are in such active practices. The days when it would be prudent to treat a patient over the phone that one has not seen in years are no longer here. Perhaps a few words about my background in 1962 might help explain how this all happened.

The years between 1950 and 1962 might be considered the "wild west days" of antimicrobial development. For better or worse, I was one of the "cowboys". Most of us had at one time or another came under the influence of Professor Maxwell Finland, a professor at the Harvard Unit at the Boston City Hospital. I was an intern there from 1947 to mid 1948. He was the inspiring pioneer in this field. After a residency and fellowship at the University of Minnesota under Dr. Wesley Spink, one of Dr. Finland's boys, I ended up in my hometown Milwaukee as a faculty member of the Marquette University Medical School and the head of the Infection Disease Control Unit at the Milwaukee County Hospital. In addition to that, in the 1950s, I was the only infectious disease specialist practicing in Milwaukee so I had the pleasure of seeing many of the cases of bacterial endocarditis in the area. In addition, in my daily rounds at the county hospital, I had the opportunity of consulting on a wide variety of bacterial infections that ended up at the county hospital. (see references in reference section).

During the fifties, a plethora of new antibiotics became available for use in antimicrobial resistant infections. Accordingly, I had the opportunity to evaluate and study Neomycin, Gentamycin, Ristocetin, Vancomycin, and Lincomycin as they became available. Institutional guidelines had not been developed at that time so if a new antimicrobial became available that might help one of our seriously ill patients, we felt free to use it. Our conscience was our guide. Informed consents were not yet in the picture. There were no conflicts of interest involved.

After Dr. Joseph Noble finished his service in the Air Force, he became and still is a respected and beloved cardiologist in Indianapolis.

CHRONOLOGICAL CORRESPONDENCE

CONTENTS OF THE APPENDIX

THE CHILDREN'S MEMORIAL HOSPITAL
707 FULLERTON AVENUE
CHICAGO 14

Office of
Willis J. Potts
Surgeon-in-chief

August 18, 1948

Dear Schnells and my little Diane,

It was very kind of you to phone and send a card.
The clouds are rolling away.

Sincerely,

Willis J. Potts

WILLIAM O. MCQUISTON, MD
ANESTHESIOLOGY
1604 West Parkside Drive
Peoria, Illinois

Dear Mrs. Schnell,

I wish to thank you for the slides of Diane. She is a beautiful girl and I hope that sometime I will be able to see her again. The Willis J. Potts Memorial Symposium on Tetralogy of Fallot was fine tribute to a great man. Drs. Kirklin and Paul showed Diane's slides starting with those in 1946 and at the end of that paper. I showed the slides which you sent me. It was the unexpected and dramatic touch that Dr. Potts used to use so well in his lectures.

Dr. Potts and I were very close and we often discussed our innermost thoughts. As you know, the child scheduled for the first Potts-Smith operation was an older child, an orphan with severe mental damage from her heart condition and she was expected to die momentarily. Mentally, she was already gone. She did not survive the operation. She was operated on the 16th, as scheduled. Diane, thus became the first on the 13th. If it had not been for Diane and the second operation had been first, Dr. Potts said he was doubtful if he would have ever tried the operation again. This is one of the reasons Diane has always been a very special baby to us. Her life gave us the courage to go on and the result was life for many hundreds of children throughout the world. Your and Mr. Schnell's bravery and faith remained with Dr. Potts until his death. We spoke of it on my last visit with the Potts.

May I wish a very special Christmas to a very special family.

Wm. O. McQuiston

THE CHILDREN'S MEMORIAL HOSPITAL
707 FULLERTON AVENUE
CHICAGO 14

OFFICE OF
Willis J. Potts
Surgeon-in-chief

December 26, 1948

Dear Mr. and Mrs. Schnell and Diane,

Thank you for the pictures. They are beautiful. It was my most appreciated Christmas gift. That little dolly is the sweetest little duffer. Again, her picture shall be framed and hung in my office with the others.

Sincerely,

Willis J. Potts

BURTON A. WAISBREN, M.D.

August 26, 1964

Dr. Harold W. Anderson
135 E. Main Street
Oyster Bay, N.Y.

Dear Dr. Anderson:

Mr. Schnell has requested that I send you a report regarding his daughter, Miss Diane Schnell. Since Dr. Waisbren is out of the office until August 28, I hope this is the information you desired.

Dr. Waisbren was first asked to see this patient while making rounds at Milwaukee County General Hospital and at the urgent request of the referring doctor, he immediately left and went to Waukesha Memorial Hospital where he found her literally dying of an acute bacterial endocarditis and staphylococcal pneumonia. During the rest of the greater part of that day, arranged for transference to St. Joseph's Hospital and instituted a therapeutic program that ultimately proved life saving.

Included in the activities on this young patient's behalf were numerous conferences with the family, referring doctor, and with Dr. Potts of Chicago, who had done the first Potts operation on her approximately 16 years ago. During her treatment, she developed exfoliative dermatitis, complicated therapeutic program to treat the endocarditis, heart failure, empyema, exfoliative dermatitis, anemia and staphylococcal pneumonia. A copy of the therapeutic program can be obtained by writing to St. Joseph's Hospital, Medical Records, 5000 W. Chambers, Milwaukee, Wisconsin.

The patient was last seen on May 31, 1963. She was on no medication at that time. There was no shortness of breath.

Her weight had been constant. She was to see Dr. Potts in a month regarding surgery.

If additional information is necessary, please feel free to call me.

Sincerely yours,

Burton A. Waisbren, M.D
Per pjr

BAW/pjr

Burton A. Waisbren, Sr.,M.D., FACP

WILLIS J. POTTS, M.D.
524 Yawl Lane
Sarasota, Florida

October 18, 1965

Dear Jane and Andy Schnell,

Thanks for your letter. I've thought about Diane so often and wondered how she was doing. The doctor didn't write me after the gallbladder operation.

You know, I've been doing a lot of thinking about Diane's condition. As you know, the deformities inside the heart can now be corrected by open-heart surgery with the aid of the pump-oxygenator. Have you given any thought to the possibility of undertaking such a procedure? It is a big operation and a bit hazardous. If successful, she could look forward to a more or less, more rather than less, normal life expectancy. Undoubtedly the endocarditis is located at the site of the aortic-pulmonary quartonaries, it is apt to flare up again. Taking down the aortoraisis and correcting the defects inside the heart would likely eliminate the possibility of recurrence of endocarditis.

I'm sure you have considered the possibility of such an operation. Diane will soon be at that age when some boy is going to look awfully attractive. There is a definite risk to the operation and I'm not advising, just offering a subject for discussion. If ever you should consider exploration of all the angels be sure to write me. There are only a few surgeons in this country I trust.

Just give Diane my love and use your judgment about any further discussion.

Sincerely,

W. Potts

Note about this letter which I found in her chart:

Apparently the Schnells wrote to Dr. Potts about the endocarditis after her acute episode in New York. He advised what was done about twenty years later. It's interesting to speculate as to what the future would have brought had Diane and her family followed Dr. Potts suggestion in 1965. I wonder what surgeon he would have chosen at that time for the operation. I was not in the loop at that time and feel badly that I was not up on her options at that time. I believe Dr. Potts had returned to Florida when he wrote this letter.

Burton A. Waisbren, Sr., M.D., FACP

DEPARTMENT OF THE AIR FORCE
2792D USAF Hospital (AFLC)
Tinker Air Force Base, Oklahoma 73145

Reply to
Attn Of: RR 25 September 1970

Subject: Mrs. Diane Pontrelli

To : Dr. John Kirklin
     Chairman, Department of Surgery
     University of Alabama Medical School
     Birmingham, Alabama

Dear Dr. Kirklin

It was my pleasure to participate with you as a member of the Guest Faculty for Dr. Hursts' "Five Days of Cardiology" last May in Atlanta and I enjoyed meeting you then. I certainly benefitted from your discussions.

I am writing you now about a favorite patient of mine, Mrs. Diane Pontrelli. I have enclosed a narrative summary of her recent hospitalization and a copy of a cardiac catheterization performed in 1968.

Briefly Mrs. Pontrelli is a 24 year-old lady with tetralogy of Fallot who was of considerable interest on several scores: (1.) she is the first patient ever to receive a Potts' anastomosis (and that, of course, performed by Dr. Potts 24 years ago), (2) she has now suffered three episodes of bacterial endocarditis (or endarteritis), (3) she is one of the first patients to receive Lincomycin for staphylococcal endocarditis, and (4) she is one of the few patients to have suffered from a gram positive rod endocarditis and certainly one of the first to be treated for this with a combination of Lincomycin and Gentamicin.

After you have had an opportunity to review her clinical course and catheterization, I would very much appreciate your considering the patient for tatal correction of tetralogy of Fallot.   I am, of course, familiar with the difficulty occasionally posed by the previous Pott's anastomosis, but do not believe, both after clinical examination and a review of her previous catheterization, that her lungs and pulmonary vasulature have suffered significantly as a result of the anastomosis.

I would appreciate your informing me of your impressions and advice. If you agree that total correction should be considered, I will arrange for the patient to visit you, preferably next spring if that time is convenient for you.

Sincerely,

R. JOE NOBLE, MAJOR, USAF, MC
Chief, Department of Internal Medicine

Burton A. Waisbren, Sr.,M.D., FACP

March 4, 1971

Dr. John Kirklin
Chairman, Department of Surgery
University of Alabama Medical School
Birmingham, Alabama

Re: Diane Pontrelli

Dear Dr. Kirklin,

This is in regard to Diane Pontrelli, the case that Dr. Noble and myself have been corresponding about in regard to the correction of the Tetralogy of Fallot, with the taking down of the original Potts operation.

I did a complete examination of Diane on March 1, 1971 and feel she is in excellent shape for the surgery. I believe you already are in receipt of the Cauterization done in 1968, The main rationale for the surgery, of course, are the three cases of Sub Bacterial Endocarditis. Diane is extremely allergic to both Penicillin and Erythromycin but tolerated the Lincomycin which we recently gave her for the last case of Endocarditis.

She is now taking 1 ½ grams of Lincomycin a day which I would continue through the surgery. If she becomes infected or there is an infectious disease problem after the surgery it would be helpful to know she can tolerate Gentamycin without allergic reaction.

I am having a blood culture drawn this week. I would assume that by the time of surgery we would have two negative blood cultures that have held for over a month.

I, of course, will look forward to your final report regarding this classic case. If I can be of any help, at any time, please call on me.

Kindest regards.

Sincerely yours,

Burton A. Waisbren, M.D.

BAW:sah

Cc: Diane Pontrelli

May 4, 1971

Dr. Milton Paul
The Children's Hospital
Chicago, Illinois

Dear Milton:

Diane Pontrelli was the first patient operated upon by Dr. Pott's for an aorto-pulmonary anastomosis. Her name at that time I believe was Miss Diane Schnell. At any rate we recently operated upon her and I am quite certain that she has the rare malformation of double outlet right ventricle. We have operated upon only one other such case. I thought you would like to have this for your records and I am enclosing a copy of the operative note and my letter to her doctor.

Warm personal regards.

Sincerely,

John W. Kirklin, M.D.
Professor and Chairman

JWK:rb
Enclosure

THE WILLIS J. POTTS CHILDREN'S HEART CENTER

The CHILDREN'S MEMORIAL HOSPITAL
2300 CHILDREN'S PLAZA
CHICAGO, ILL 60614   May 20, 1971
312 348-4040

Burton A. Waisbren, M.D.
Suite 616 Bankers Building
203 East Wisconsin Avenue
Milwaukee, Wisconsin 53202   Re: Diane Pontrelli
                                     nee: Schnell

Dear Dr. Waisbren:

Dr. Kirklin sent us a copy of Diane's operative report of the
surgery he performed in Birmingham on 4-14-71, also a copy
of the letter addressed to you.

As you know Diane Pontrelli was operated on here at Children's
Memorial Hospital by Dr. Potts in 1946. We would appreciate
it very much to receive any information of catheterization done
prior to surgery and/or any other pertinent data that you could
send us concerning past treatment. We assume you know
Diane was the first patient operated by Dr. Potts for an aorto-
pulmonary anastomosis and is of special interest to us. Please
also keep us informed of her future progress.

Sincerely Yours,

Roger B. Cole, M.D.
Division of Cardiology

RBC:gh

Burton A. Waisbren, Sr.,M.D., FACP

the University of Alabama in Birmingham / 1919 SEVENTH AVENUE
SOUTH/BIRMINGHAM ALABAMA 35233

the **Medical** *Center* / **DEPARTMENT OF SURGERY**

May 4, 1971

Burton A. Waisbren, M.D.
Suite 616 Bankers Building
203 East Wisconsin Avenue
Milwaukee, Wisconsin 53202

Dear Dr. Waisbren:

We were really surprised in the case of Diane Pontrelli to find the very unusual condition of double outlet left ventricle with severe pulmonary stenosis. I am quite certain that this is the anatomic diagnosis although we did not identify it as such in our preoperative angiographic studies. I am enclosing a copy of the operative note.

Diane got along very nicely postoperatively and indeed her postoperative course was quite without complications. Her only real problem was a little continuing hoarseness due to the endotracheal tube. She was on no medications at the time of dismissal.

At the time of dismissal we heard a grade II ejection murmur along the left sterna boarder and no diastolic murmur. There was no evidence of fluid retention. Her heart rate was 88 beats per minute and she was in sinus rhythm. We did suggest a 0.5 gram sodium diet for three more weeks and then after that we felt she could pretty much do as she wished. We do hope you will let us hear from you from time to time.

Sincerely,

John W. Kirklin, M.D.
Professor and Chairman

JWK:rb
Cc: Dr. Milton Paul

the University of Alabama in Birmingham / 1919 SEVENTH AVENUE
SOUTH/BIRMINGHAM ALABAMA 35233

*the **Medical** Center* / **DEPARTMENT OF SURGERY**

January 4, 1974

Mr. and Mrs. Andrew Schnell, Jr.
849 Ridgewood Drive
Waukesha, Wisconsin 53186

Dear Mr. and Mrs. Schnell:

Thank you so much for thinking of me at Christmas-time. It was
very kind of you to send me a Christmas card and I appreciate it
very much.

We are delighted that Diane continues to do so well and appreciate
hearing from you
from time to time.

We all send best wishes to you for a wonderful New Year.

Sincerely,

John W. Kirklin, M.D.
Professor and Chairman

/mm

September 30, 1975

Mrs. Steve Cummings
804 Lincoln Avenue
Waukesha, Wisconsin 53186

Dear Mrs. Cummings:

I am so sorry that I missed seeing you when you were here in August but I know Dr. Stockinger talked with you in some detail. Also I have corresponded with your father and with Dr. Waisbren about you.

As you know we do feel that the new passageway we made between the heart and the pulmonary artery has probably become compressed and narrowed and is beginning to cause you real trouble. We think that we should do another cardiac catheterization in order to prove whether this is the case or not. If it is then another operation should be done to replace this tube with a new one in a more appropriate position. *I know that since you have just recently married, you must not look upon such an undertaking with much favor.* However, I do think it is important for you and I do think the chances are very good that it will work out just perfectly.

I wish that we could do your operation sooner but the first definitely available date, since your problem does not seem to be an emergency is Monday, the 8th of December. I am asking my associate, Dr. William Baxley, to plan your cardiac catheterization for Friday, the 5th of December. We would like for you to come into the hospital on my surgical service on Wednesday, the 3rd of December.

We do look forward very much to seeing you and we certainly will do our level best to be sure that everything works out well for you.

Sincerely,

John W. Kirklin, M.D.
Professor and Chairman

JWK:js
Enclosures
Cc: Dr. William Baxley
      Dr. Burton Waisbren

Burton A. Waisbren, Sr.,M.D., FACP

CARDIOVASCULAR PHYSICIANS, LTD.
2040 WEST WISCONSIN AVENUE. Suite 707   /
Milwaukee, Wisconsin 53233   /   342-8700
BURTON J. FRIEDMAN, M.D.,   Donald
A. SPRING, M.D., F.A.C.C.

December 27, 1976

Burton Waisbren, M.D.
700 North Water Street
Milwaukee, Wisconsin 53202

RE: Diane Cummings

Dear Bud:

This patient is in final month of pregnancy and has no complaints.

The chest is clear. Right ventricular heave is noted. A second sound in the pulmonic area is palpable and there is a loud ejection systolic murmur at the left sterna border with wide splitting of the second heart sound, both on inspiration and expiration. No diastolic murmurs are heard. No left ventricular heave, no cyanosis, no edema.

The patient looks wonderful and I see no problem with her delivery. I would suggest that she will have to be covered by antibiotics at the time of her delivery.

Very truly yours,

Burton J. Friedman, M.D.

BJF:llh
Cc: James J. Nocon, M.D.

This note was written in a congratulations card:

Dear Mr. and Mrs. Schnell

Thank you for sharing the almost unbelievable and happy news of Jeffery Allan's birth with me. Your letter, with the news paper article, arrived on the eve of my retirement, which I look forward to with mixed emotions. It helped tremendously to cheer me up.

A day or two after Diane's operation on Friday, Sept. 13th, 1946, Dr. Carlson, the famous University of Chicago physiologist, a teacher, and a great friend of Dr. Potts visited Children's Memorial to see Diane. As the three of us stood by her crib, Dr. Carlson said "You are a historic baby." I cannot think of a better description of Jeffery than the one you used, "this miracle baby."

Dr. Potts and I always believed God was very close to us in the operating room and sometimes as I drove out to Oak Park to spend the night with the Potts, he would say "God held us by the hand today." I believe the spirits of Dr. Potts, Dr. Smith and Dr. Gibson are watching over the Schnells and the Cummings and they would want to join me in congratulations to two very brave and special families and to say God Bless You All.

Dr. McQuiston
1977

Burton A. Waisbren, Sr.,M.D., FACP

WAISBREN CLINIC
BURTON A. WAISBREN

INTERNAL MEDICINE
INFECTIOUS DISEASES
ONCOLOGY
IMMUNOMOCULATION THERAPY

2315 NORTH LAKE DRIVE, SETON TOWER, SUITE
815, MILWAUKEE, WISCONSIN 53211
TELEPHONE (414) 272-1929

December 3, 1992

Cardiovascular Service
Medical Center
University of Alabama
Birmingham, AL

Attention: Dr. Kirkland or his successor

Dear Sirs:

I have enclosed a brief update regarding Mrs. Cummings who was operated on by your staff some years ago. There were two operations done, and after this she got along very well until just last month, at which time she went into heart failure. I'm not sure that she didn't go into heart failure because of lack of compliance and also because of the increase in sodium in her diet. The cardiologists who've seen her here have suggested that she have another catheterization based upon what has happened, and both Diane and I feel that should she need a catheterization or further surgery that perhaps it should be done at your service since you are aware of what went on at the first two operations. I've enclosed the consultation of Dr. Slosky, a very fine cardiologist here in Milwaukee, and the recent echo reports, and we would appreciate hearing from you in regard to what we should do.

If you feel that no matter what the findings are that further heart surgery is counter indicated, we will handle the matter here. If on the other hand you feel that another operation might be indicated, then I would rather have her evaluated by you with catheterization and an opinion. Your help and consideration regarding this very interesting case will be deeply appreciated.

It's not been 35 years since Dr. Potts did her original operation, and we hope that Diane can have another good period of life utilizing state-of-the-art cardiovascular repairs.

Kindest regards.

Sincerely yours,

Burton A. Waisbren, Sr., M.D.

Burton A. Waisbren, Sr., M.D., FACP

UAB SCHOOL OF
MEDICINE
Department of Surgery
Division of Cardiothoracic Surgery

February 2, 1993

Diane Cummings
804 Lincoln
Waukesha, WI   53186

Dear Ms. Cummings:

We are all very pleased with your excellent recovery after your recent major open heart operation. As you know, we replaced your severely stenotic conduit with a new homograft valve extracardiac conduit, and your heart tolerated the operation very nicely. We are all hopeful that you can get along very nicely from this operation for many years.

You should contact Dr. Waisbren upon your return home so that you might gradually increase your activities over the next six to eight weeks under his guidance. Please avoid any heavy lifting for at least two months.

We certainly have enjoyed caring for you, and if you have any questions or problems related to your operation, please do not hesitate to call upon us. We would very much like to hear from you from time to time regarding your progress.

With best wishes.

Sincerely,

James K. Kirklin, M.D.
Professor of Surgery
Division of Cardiothoracic Surgery

JKK.wph
Cc: Burton A. Waisbren, Sr., M.D.
    John W. Kirklin, M.D.
    Sharon Dailey, M.D.

The University of Alabama at Birmingham
739 Zeigler Research Building / 703 South 19th Street
Birmingham, Alabama 35294-0007 / (205) 934-3368 / (205) 934-5261

Burton A. Waisbren, Sr.,M.D., FACP

February 14, 2007

To: Cummings Family/Schnell Family

Dear Stephen and Families,

Please accept my condolences on the passing onward of Diane. I only know of her from stories from my parents, Dr Martin and Elsie Werra. But what stories they were. She influenced my father in his work and me in mine as a family physician and a storyteller to my children and grandchildren. My daughter in grade school won the Science Fair with her clay models of congenital heart disease including Tetralogy of Fallot, etc., including transposition of the aorta. She went on and became a surgeon and was chosen after being Chief Surgical Resident at Kaiser in San Francisco to go on to a fellowship in Heart Surgery in Texas to then become the Heart Surgeon for Kaiser Hospital in San Francisco. She almost did it but decided a family came first and came back to Ukiah and settled down having 3 children and specializing in breast cancer surgery. As a family physician, one major endeavor I did was fighting to preserve the use of abandoned dogs scheduled to be euthanized at the pound to instead be used at University of California San Francisco Medical School for developing medicine and surgery, knowing they could be models for new heart procedures and new heart surgeons. We won the battle. Interestingly, my surgeon daughter's baby, Julie, was diagnosed at birth with transposition of the great vessels, was operated on and saved at UCSF by a surgeon who practiced the procedure on dogs from our pound. Julia is now 10 and is a star of her basketball team. This comes from the legacy of the Schnells and Diane.

I enclose an e-mail I sent to my Werra relative when my cousin Jude Werra (who heard Dad's story) saw the newspapers' account of Diane's obituary and notified me.

I have a cigarette lighter the Schnell's gave my Dad from Diane, memorializing her surgery and first walking. I suspect this memento would be better kept in your family. Please let me know if you would like it, and I will send it on.

Sincerely,

Bob Werra

REFERENCES

1. Murphy JG, Gersh BJ, Mair DD, Fuster V, McGoon MD, Ilstrup DM, McGoon DC, Kirklin JW, Danielson GK. Long-term Outcome in Patients Undergoing Surgical Repair of Tetralogy of Fallot. 329:593-599; 1993.

2. Cole RB, Muster AJ, Fixler DE, Paul MH. Long-term Results of Aortapulmonary Anastomosis for Tetralogy of Fallot: Morbidity and Mortality, 1946-1969. Circulation 1971;43:263-271.

3. Morales DLS, Braud BE, Gunter KS, Carberry KE, Arrington KA, Heinle JS, McKenzie ED, Fraser CD Jr (2006). Encouraging Results for the Contegra Conduit in the Problematic Right Ventricle-to-Pulmonary Artery Connection. *J. Thorac. Cardiovasc. Surg.* 132:665-671.

4. Horer J, Friebe J, Schreiber C, Kostolny M, Cleuzios J, Holper K, Lange R (2005). Correction of Tetralogy of Fallot and of Pulmonary Atresia with Ventricular Septal Defect in Adults. *Ann. Thorac. Surg.* 80:2285-2291.

5. Hekmat M, Rafieyian S, Foroughi M, Majidi Tehrani MM, Beheshti MM, Hassantash SA (2005). Associated Coronary Anomalies in135 Iranian Patients with Tetralogy of Fallot. *Asian Cardiovasc. Thorac. Ann.* 13_307-310.

6. Veldtman GR, Connolly HM, Grogan M, Ammash NM, Warnes CA (2004). Outcomes of Pregnancy in Women with Tetralogy of Fallot. *J Am Coll Cardiol* 44:174-180.

7. Ghai A, Silversides C, Harris L, Webb GD, Siu SC, Therrien J (2002). Left Ventricular Dysfunction is a Risk Factor for Sudden Cardiac Death in Adults Later after Repair of Tetralogy of Fallot. *J Am Coll Cardiol* 40:1675-1680.

8. Discigil B, Dearani JA, Puga FJ, Schaff HV, Hagler DJ, Warnes CA, Danielson GK (2001). Late Pulmonary Valve Replacement

after Repair of Tetralogy of Fallot. *J Thorac. Cardiovasc. Surg.* 121:0344-351.

9. Oechslin EN, Harrison DA, Harris L, Downar E, Webb GD, Sui SS, Williams WG (1999). Reoperation in Adults with Repair of Tetralogy of Fallot: Indications and Outcomes. *J Thorac. Cardiovasc. Surg.* 118:245-251.

10. Cerfolio RJ, Danielson GK, Warnes CA, Puga FJ, Schaff HV, Anderson BJ, Ilstrup DM (1995). Results of an Autologous Tissue Reconstruction for Replacement of Obstructed Extracardiac Conduits. *J Thorac. Cardiovasc. Surg.* 110:1359-1368.

11. Rosenthal A (1993). Adults with Tetralogy of Fallot – Repaired, Yes; Cured, No. *NEJM* 329:655-656.

12. Waisbren BA. Experiences with the New Antibiotic Gentamicin. 119:518-527; 1969.

13. Blalock A, Taussig HB. The Blalock-Taussig-Thomas Collaboration: A Model for Medical Progress. 128(3):189-202; 1945.

14. Blalock A, Taussig HB. The Surgical Treatment of Malformations of the Heart in Which There is :Pulmonary Stenosis or Pulmonary Atresia. 251:2123-2137; 1984.

15. Waisbren BA. In Vitro Activity Against Micrococcus Pyogenes of Various Combinations of Antimicrobial Agents. 46:483-591; 1955.

16. Waisbren BA, Spink WW. A Clinical Appraisal of Neomycin, Ann. Int. Med. 33:1099-1119; 1950.

17. Waisbren BA, Carr C. Penicillin and Chloramphenicol in the Treatment of Infections Dueto Proteus Organisms, Am. J. Med. Sci. 223: 418-421; 1952.

18. Waisbren BA. Lincomycin in Larger Doses. 206:2118; 1968.

19. De Ycaza MM, Waisbren BA, Goodman JS. Therapy of Bacterial endocarditis in Penicillin-Hypersensitive Patients: Two Cases Treated with Lincomycin and Streptomycin. 120:361-364; 1967.

20. Waisbren BA. Comparative Clinical Effectiveness and Toxicity of Vancomycin, Ristocetin, and Kanamycin, *Arch Intern Med.* 106:179-193; 1960.

21. Waisbren BA. The Combination of Erythromycin and Chlortetracycline for the Treatment of Bacterial Endocarditis. 44:945; 1954.

22. Waisbren BA, Hastings EV. Bacterial Endocarditis Due to Pseudomonas Aeruginosa. 55:218-222; 1953.

23. Oosterhof T, Jacobs M, Cramer MJ, Mjulder BJM. Survival into Seventh Decade after a Potts Palliation for Tetralogy of Fallot. 2:55-57; 2007.

24. Waisbren BA. Antibiotic Treatment of Bacterial Endocarditis due to Enterococcus. 94:846-852; 1954.

25. Finland M. Treatment of Bacterial Endocarditis: Dosage of Penicillin, Use of Other Antibiotics and Treatment of Patients with Negative Blood Cultures. 9:292-299; 1954.

26. Waisbren BA, Carr C, Dunnette J. The Tube Dilution Method of Determining Bacterial Sensitivity to Antibiotics, J. Clin. Path. 21:884-891; 1951.

27. Busch UW, Mathur VS, Garcia E, Cooley DA, de Castro CM, Hall RJ. Late Deterioration in Tetralogy of Fallot: Unusual Findings and Successful Correction. 138(9):1423-1424; 1978.

28. Cooley DA. In Memoriam John W. Kirklin 1917-2004. 31(2):113; 2004.

29. Cole RB, Muster AJ, Fixler DE, Paul MH. Long-term Results of Aortopulmonary Anastomosis for Tetralogy of Fallot: Morbidity and Mortality, 1946-1969. 43:263; 1971.